DOCTOR'S LITTLE BOOK OF ANSWERS

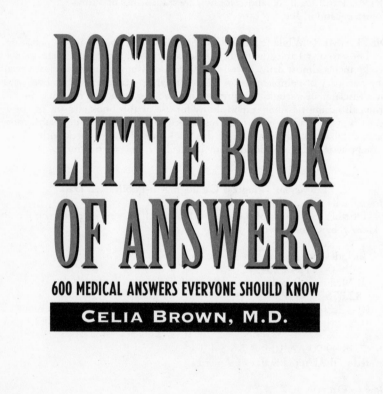

DOCTOR'S LITTLE BOOK OF ANSWERS

600 MEDICAL ANSWERS EVERYONE SHOULD KNOW

CELIA BROWN, M.D.

PRIMA PUBLISHING

PRIMA PUBLISHING and colophon are trademarks of Prima
Communications, Inc.

DISCLAIMER: While Prima Publishing believes the sources used in creating
this book to be reliable, the medical field is rapidly changing and there are new
developments almost daily. Therefore, Prima Publishing cannot guarantee accu-
racy, adequacy or completeness of the information contained in this book and
must disclaim all warranties, express or implied, regarding the information.
Prima also cannot assume responsibility for use of this book and any use by a
reader is at the reader's own risk. This book is not intended to be a substitute
for medical advice, and any user of this book should always check with a licensed physician before adopting any particular course of treatment.

Library of Congress Cataloging-in-Publication Data
Brown, Celia.
    Doctor's little book of answers : 600 medical answers everyone should
know / by Celia Brown.
        p.   cm.
    Includes index.
    ISBN 0-7615-0325-0
    I. Medicine, Popular—Miscellanea. I. Title.
RC82.B76 1995
610—dc20   95-39609
                                                                CIP

96 97 98 99 00 AA 10 9 8 7 6 5 4 3
Printed in the United States of America

How to Order:
Single copies may be ordered from Prima Publishing, P.O. Box 1260BK,
Rocklin, CA 95677; telephone (916) 632-4400. Quantity discounts are also
available. On your letterhead, include information concerning the intended use
of the books and the number of books you wish to purchase.

For my father

Legend

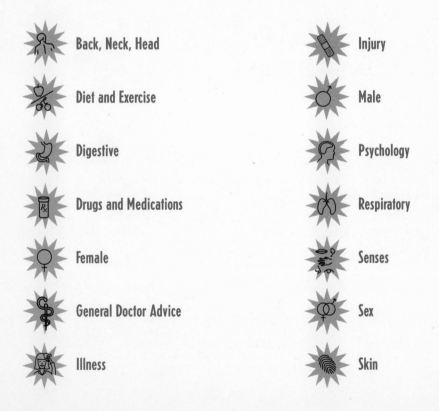

Back, Neck, Head

Diet and Exercise

Digestive

Drugs and Medications

Female

General Doctor Advice

Illness

Injury

Male

Psychology

Respiratory

Senses

Sex

Skin

Author's Note

This book is a consumer's guide to basic medicine. It describes some simple things that will help you stay well. It also suggests tricks that will make you feel better when you are sick. This book offers guidelines about *when* to see your doctor and *when to* stay home. Some of the problems that may send you to the emergency room can easily wait until the next day, but some problems can't. If you know the difference, you can save yourself a long wait, a big hassle, and a lot of money.

This book will tell you what is really in brand-name medicines, and how to buy the same ingredients for a fraction of the price. All the medicines are listed in the glossary in the back of the book. Use it and save your hard-earned dollars.

Acknowledgments

My sincerest thanks go to those people who helped me write this book: Dr. Jane Butlin, Dr. Robin Schoenthaler, Mark Sickorez, R.Ph., my uncle Marvin Holen, the participants of the Love and Power Workshop on Isla Mujeres March 1993, and mostly my husband Dr. Glen Sickorez, without whose help I couldn't have done it.

DOCTOR'S LITTLE BOOK OF ANSWERS

1

Everyone needs a doctor. Even if you never get sick, you still need a doctor. There are plenty of things you can do to stay well. Pick a doctor you like and feel you can talk to.

2

When you are sick always drink plenty of clear fluids.

3

All medicines have generic names. A generic name is the real name of the drug. For example, Benadryl is simply a brand name and diphenhydramine is the real, generic name of the drug. They are the same drug with different names. Drugs sold under their generic names are always cheaper than the corresponding name brands. Use generics!

4

Buy a thermometer and use it!

When should I go to the emergency room after a bee sting?

If you have any trouble breathing (call an ambulance)

If you have hives all over your body

If you have a history of serious allergy to bee stings

5

A lcohol doesn't kill germs.

6

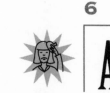

A llergies *itch!* Infections *hurt!*

7

S ome people have bowel movements three times a day; some people have them every three days. There is a wide range of what's normal. If your normal pattern *changes,* see your doctor.

8

Y ou can't catch an ear infection.

9

D o not blindly trust health insurance companies. They are interested in profits, not your health.

2

10

Nausea is horrible. It usually means that your body is unhappy for some reason. Try to find out why.

11

A primary care doctor is a general doctor who oversees and can coordinate all your medical care. He or she will send you to a specialist if necessary. If you are sick, make sure you call you primary care doctor first!

12

A normal temperature is between 97.5 and 100 degrees Fahrenheit. Everyone's temperature is lower in the morning and goes up slightly in the late afternoon.

13

Lips can sunburn. If they do, keep something on them constantly. They will heal, but it can take quite awhile. If they keep bothering you, see a skin doctor.

14

If you don't have a doctor, *shop* for one! It's at least as important as having a good hairdresser or plumber.

When should I go to the emergency room after a bite?

If you've been bitten by a person

If the bite is on your hand or needs stitches

If you were bitten by a wild animal

15

If you get your penis or scrotum caught in a zipper, cut the *bottom* of the *zipper* open with scissors and it will separate easily.

16

Smoking is *terrible* for your body. It is just about the worst thing you can do. Quit! You'll save a lot of money and live longer.

17

If you are hit in the eye and suddenly lose your sight, have someone drive you to an eye doctor or the emergency room immediately!

18

Some medicines can cause heartburn if you don't take them with plenty of water. Swallow *all* pills with a whole glass of water and wait before you lie down.

19

It takes about thirty minutes for sunscreen to soak in and work. Put it on *before* you go into the sun.

20

Tylenol is the name brand for acetaminophen. Acetaminophen is the generic, real name. Don't be frightened by all those letters. Acetaminophen is the ingredient in most "non-aspirin" pain relievers. It's good for pain relief and fever, and it's easy on the stomach.

21

If your pain keeps you up at night, see your doctor in the morning.

22

Creams like Icy Hot or Ben Gay only numb the skin. Don't waste your money on them.

23

A virus is a germ that causes many different kinds of infections. For example, viruses cause colds, flu, and AIDS. For the most part, we cannot cure these viral diseases using antibiotics.

24

Bacteria are germs that cause different kinds of infections. Examples of bacterial infections are strep throat, urinary tract infections, and gonorrhea. We generally can cure illness caused by bacteria using antibiotics.

25

Bacteria cause diseases that we *can* cure, and viruses cause diseases that we generally *cannot* cure. Most minor colds and flu are caused by viruses. This is the reason antibiotics (they kill bacteria) are useless against minor viral infections such as colds and flu.

26

Gargling will make your sore throat worse. Don't do it!

27

If you're into the new Rollerblade craze, wear *all* the protective gear. It's expensive, but not as expensive as a broken wrist!

28

Medicine is not really an exact science where there are clear right and wrong answers. That's why when you leave your doctor's office you sometimes feel frustrated because you're not really sure what's wrong with you. This is usually because your doctor isn't really sure, either. This doesn't mean your doctor is bad. She is simply telling you the truth.

29

Motrin, Advil, and Nuprin are just brand names for ibuprofen. The generic is just as good as the name brand. A solid dose is 400 to 600 milligrams, taken three times a day. Make sure to take it with food. If it hurts your stomach, stop taking it!

30

Minor injuries or irritations to the penis usually happen because you are allergic to something you are using during sex. Spermicidal foam is one common culprit.

31

Calcium is very important for women. If you are older than eighteen you should get at least 1,200 milligrams per day. It's hard to get this from your diet, so take a drugstore brand calcium supplement before bed.

32

If you find a lump in your breast, checking it constantly until you get to the doctor can make it really sore.

33

If you have a sprain, bruise, or any other injury, most of the pain you feel is from swelling. The sooner you ice and elevate the sprain, the less it will hurt.

34

If your doctor orders a test on you, ask "Will the results of this test change the treatment?" If he says no, ask why he is ordering the test. If he can't explain exactly why, it's fair to suspect he either can't figure out what's wrong with you, or he is afraid of getting sued.

35

Always urinate after having sex. This may prevent urinary tract infections, especially if you are a woman.

36

A fever over 101 degrees is considered significant for an adult. Don't worry too much about a fever under 101 degrees.

37

Acetaminophen (sold under the brand name Tylenol) can be a dangerous drug if you take an overdose. Nothing will happen for a few days, but if you don't see a doctor soon and tell her, the resulting irreversible liver damage is often fatal.

38

If you have indigestion frequently or wake up in the middle of the night with heartburn or pain in the upper part of your belly, it's probably stomach irritation. To remedy this you should cut out caffeine, alcohol, cigarettes, and ibuprofen and stop eating just before bed.

39

We used to think that suffering built character. It doesn't! Pain actually damages your body's ability to deal with stress. If your pain keeps you up at night and it won't go away with over-the-counter medicines, see your doctor.

40

If you need a sterilized needle, hold a needle in a flame until it glows red, then dip it in povidone—iodine (you can buy this at the drugstore). Don't burn yourself; wait until the needle cools before using it.

If you are a woman over fifty, you should have a mammogram every year.

Chicken pox is a *very* contagious virus. It is contagious until all the blisters have dried up. If you haven't had the disease or taken the new vaccine, and you do get exposed, plan on getting sick. Adults often get sicker than children. Don't scratch the sores. Take diphenhydramine, which is the generic name for Benadryl. Use acetaminophen, and take oatmeal or Aveeno baths. Try Burrows solution from the pharmacy; you don't need a prescription. Stock up on some good books and movies. *Do not leave your house* while you are contagious.

Breathe through your nose if possible. All those little nose hairs have a purpose—they're filters. Your mouth doesn't have them.

44

Everyone should have a primary care doctor. Ask friends about their doctors if you don't know one. When you get a name, call and ask how long the wait is for a regular appointment. "New Patient" appointments often take longer to get because they take more of the doctor's time. If the time it takes to get a regular appointment is more than one week, look for another doctor.

45

Nonprescription asthma inhalers don't work very well and can be dangerous. Don't waste your money.

46

Use condoms. They are the cheapest health insurance you can buy.

47

Drug companies are trying to make a profit. Their labels are intended to sell their products. There are only a small amount of actual drugs in all those medicines, and they are almost all generic. Read the labels and use the glossary in the back of this book.

How should I take care of a pulled muscle?

Use ice on it as soon as possible and as often as possible

Never use heat on it

Rest the muscle until it stops hurting

48

If you have strained your neck and back in a car accident, the pain will probably get worse over the first three days.

49

Pain medicines that claim to be great for headaches just have added caffeine. (See tip 47.) If you have a headache, use a generic pain drug and drink some coffee; it's much cheaper!

50

You can have a sexually transmitted disease and not know it, especially if you are a woman. If you are sexually active and don't always use condoms, see your doctor regularly and ask her to take cultures for the most common diseases: gonorrhea and chlamydia.

51

If your skin has a scaly, itchy rash that comes and goes, the best treatment is *not to scratch*.

52

Walk with your shoulders back, your chest out, and your belly in. Good posture can help with back problems, and it also makes you feel better.

53

If you burn yourself, immediately run cold water over the burn for ten minutes.

54

If you are over thirty-five, it feels as if it's almost impossible to lose weight. This is because your metabolism really starts to slow down as you get older. Exercise is the key. Eating less fat and really increasing your exercise is the only way!

55

If you're prone to alcohol hangovers, drink three large glasses of water, take two ibuprofen before you go to bed, and sleep for as long as possible.

What should I do for a headache?

Drink some coffee and take acetaminophen

Ice and massage your neck and scalp

56

To stop a nosebleed, sit up, put tissue to your nose, and press your index finger over the length of your nose. Keep it there *without moving your finger* for ten minutes. Don't blow your nose for at least eight hours.

57

If your doctor gives you a new prescription, especially if you have to pay for your own medications, ask the pharmacist to give you just enough for a week. That way if it doesn't work or if you have a side effect, you won't be stuck with a bottle full of useless pills.

58

If you suddenly get terrible pain in your big toe and it's red and warm, you may have gout. It's not an emergency but see your doctor. In the meantime try ice, ibuprofen, and elevation.

59

If you have a discharge from the end of your penis, see your doctor.

60

If your sex partner has a discharge from his penis, see your doctor.

61

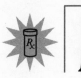

Always read the labels on drugstore medicines.

62

If your skin gets scaly, red, and itchy from time to time, it's probably some kind of eczema. Don't scratch; use lubricating lotions right after bathing and try hydrocortisone 10 (1 percent hydrocortisone) cream from the drugstore. If this doesn't work, see your doctor.

63

If you have high blood pressure, there are some things you can do to lower it yourself. Exercise regularly, cut down on salty foods, stop smoking, cut down on alcohol, and relax! If these things don't help, see your doctor.

64

If you feel as though you must urinate constantly, have a burning pain when you do go, and sometimes only a few drops come out, you probably have a urinary tract infection. See your doctor.

65

Ice is very useful for sprains and all types of swelling. Put it on for twenty minutes, then remove it for twenty minutes. Repeat this often and never put ice directly on the skin. Frozen bags of corn or peas work well for this. They fit over the injury and can be refrozen and reused. Put the bag into a pillowcase and use an elastic bandage to hold the ice pack in place.

66

If you notice your heart jumps occasionally, don't worry, it's a normal skip called a PVC (premature ventricular contraction).

67

Laughing is good for you, especially if you're sick.

68

Cold sores on the lips are caused by a virus and worsened by the sun. You can spread them to other places on your body. Try not to touch them, wash your hands frequently, and ask your pharmacist to recommend an ointment.

69

Hospitals are businesses out to make a profit. Don't forget that when you deal with them. Check your bill, insist on good service, and remember: They need your business.

70

If you suddenly get the unquestionably worst headache of your life, go to the emergency room immediately! This could be a symptom of bleeding in the brain, which sometimes is fatal.

71

Always, always finish your antibiotics, even if you begin to feel better. The bacteria you are trying to kill don't know that you feel better and may decide to hang around.

72

It's a good idea to keep activated charcoal in the house *instead* of ipecac (the stuff that makes you vomit). If someone swallows something poisonous, administer a dose of charcoal right away and go to the emergency room immediately.

73

Douching is terrible for you. It's not only unnecessary but can cause pelvic inflammatory disease, a major cause of infertility. Don't douche.

74

In general, the signs of infection are increasing warmth, redness, swelling, pain, and pus.

75

If you are a woman, examine your breasts every month. Do this in the middle of your menstrual cycle, standing in the shower, with a soapy hand. If you notice a lump that is new or unusual, see your doctor.

76

If you have indigestion in the middle of the night, try putting six-inch high blocks under the head of your bed. If this doesn't work, see your doctor.

77

It's very common to be allergic to the metal in pierced earrings; your ears will get warm and tender to touch. Try the "allergy-free" earrings sold in accessory stores.

78

Even ten minutes of exercise is worth it. Do jumping jacks, run in place, or go up and down your stairs. Even five minutes will increase your metabolic rate enough to burn a few extra calories.

79

Doctor's don't do teeth; we skipped them in medical school. If you have a toothache, see your dentist.

80

Burns that don't blister are not a big deal. After running cold water over your burn, cut an onion and rub the fresh juice onto the burn for about an hour. This will prevent pain and blistering. It really works.

81

If you feel dizzy when you stand up suddenly, this may mean you haven't been drinking enough fluids. If you are still dizzy after you've had lots of water, see your doctor.

82

Generic drugs usually have a "drugstore" type label on them like CVS, Wal-Mart, or Thrifty.

83

If your hands get red, scaly, and itchy frequently, you may be allergic to something you put your hands in every day. This condition is common among hairdressers and dishwashers. Wear gloves and see your doctor if it won't go away.

84

When you get your blood pressure taken, check the bottom number. If it's always over ninety, see your doctor.

85

The best thing for washing out cuts is povidone–iodine in a 10 percent solution. You can get this at the drugstore. Buy the generic brand!

86

Douching does *not* prevent pregnancy.

87

If your nose runs constantly and your throat and eyes are always itchy, see an allergist; she can help.

88

All antacids do the same thing; buy the generic. If your heartburn still bothers you, see your doctor.

89

As long as it's safe, sex is good for everyone; it's free and lowfat.

When should I go to the emergency room for stitches?

If the cut is through your skin and gaping open

If the cut is bleeding so much you can't stop it with direct pressure

If the cut is over a joint and gaping open

If you can't move the area in the same way you could before getting cut

If you have any numbness that you didn't have before

If there is any chance you have something in the cut

90

Acetaminophen is often an ingredient in cold remedies. Make sure the total amount of this drug from all medicines you take is never more than 4,000 milligrams in one 24-hour period.

91

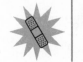

If you hurt your ankle, use ice right away. Lie on the couch with your foot up on the back of the couch. This elevates your foot above your heart, which reduces swelling. Take some pain medicine; sprained ankles hurt. Get an X-ray if you think it might be broken. Go through the same routine for other foot injuries.

92

If you have trouble sleeping, don't drink caffeinated drinks after 2:00 in the afternoon, don't drink alcohol, exercise earlier in the day, and don't worry about how much sleep you are missing.

93

No matter what kind of cut or scrape you have, it's very important to get the dirt and gravel out of it. It usually hurts, but it's worth it because dirt causes infection and scars!

94

Bronchitis is a cough that lasts. It often follows a cold. If you are younger than sixty and don't smoke, don't worry. Most of the time it's caused by a virus and can't be cured by medicine. It often hangs on for a month or more. If you smoke, are older than sixty, have a fever with the cough, or you've had it more than two weeks, see your doctor.

95

If you have unprotected sex with someone other than your regular sex partner, see your doctor and get antibiotics for gonorrhea and chlamydia. Do this before you have sex with your regular partner or both of you could be in real trouble.

96

If your feet are bothering you, ask your doctor what to do. She might not know, but give her a chance. Then see a podiatrist.

97

If the skin on the back of your upper arms and buttocks is bumpy, don't use rough skin sponges and drying soaps. They will make it worse. Use moisturizing creams and ask your doctor for some Lac-Hydrin 12 percent cream if it really bothers you.

When should I go to the emergency room with a skin infection (red, warm, tender area)?

If it is on your hand or face

If there are red streaks coming from the infected area

If you are a diabetic, especially if the infection is on your foot

If your immune system isn't working normally (for example, if you are undergoing chemotherapy or taking steroids)

98

Elevate a burn if possible; the swelling will go down, and it will hurt less.

99

Most of the expense of health care comes from procedures such as X-rays or surgeries, not from doctor visits. Talk to your doctor about your problem before having a procedure performed: It's cheaper and much less risky for you.

100

If milk and ice cream give you gas or diarrhea, you probably have lactose (milk sugar) intolerance. This bothers about fifty million people in the United States.

101

In order to digest milk sugar, or lactose, you need a natural chemical called lactase. If you have a problem with this, take pills that contain this substance when you eat dairy products, so you won't have gas or get bloated. Lactaid and Dairy Ease are brand names for the pills that contain this substance. Your drugstore probably has its own generic brand. Use it, it's half the price.

102

If you are lactose intolerant you can buy special milk that is much easier to digest. It doesn't taste exactly the same, but most women need the calcium in dairy products for healthy bones.

103

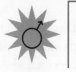

If you are male, examine your testicles every month. Do this in the shower while your hand is soapy. If you find any lumps, see your doctor.

104

Hypertension is just another word for high blood pressure.

105

If you are sick and feel like staying in bed, stay in bed! Your body knows what to do; listen to it.

106

Sprained ankles are nasty injuries because the ligaments that hold the ankle together are strained. They can take up to six weeks to heal and often feel stiff for six months.

107

If you have a cold, wash your hands frequently. Viruses stick to your hands, and you can give them to others.

108

The only people who need a flu shot are those who spend a lot of time with sick people, have heart or lung problems, or are older than sixty.

109

Don't use the nasal sprays that you can buy without a prescription. If you were to use them for longer than forty-eight hours, you'd get so addicted that you wouldn't be able to breath out of your nose at all.

110

Don't drink alcohol on an airplane; it makes you feel bad for lots of reasons.

111

One of the best times to exercise is when you feel the least energetic. If it takes you a long time to wake up, exercise in the morning and by the time you're awake, you'll be done with your workout. If you feel low in the afternoon, exercise then, you'll feel better.

112

If you have frequent, unwelcome, or disturbing thoughts that really bother you, see a psycho-therapist.

113

One glass of red wine a day may help you to live longer. We don't know if it's the alcohol or the grapes themselves. It can't hurt to drink a glass of grape juice every day if you hate wine.

114

If you need crutches, consider renting them. That should cost you about five dollars a week, much less than buying them from an emergency room or your doctor. Most medical supply places rent them. If you can't handle crutches rent a walker; they work too.

Genital herpes is a sexually transmitted disease that is caused by a virus. Once you get it, the virus never really goes away. It hangs out in your nerves and emerges to bother you whenever it wants. The first sign is a group of painful blisters on your genital area. They really hurt! If you've never had this before, don't have sex and see your doctor as soon as possible. If you have had it before, you still shouldn't have sex until all the blisters are completely cleared up. There is no good treatment for herpes; it's a virus.

Mononucleosis or "mono" is caused by a virus. There is no cure. People who have mono feel tired and sleepy all the time, and usually have a nasty sore throat. You can get it only once. If you suspect you have mono and you play any type of contact sports, stop immediately and see your doctor.

Acetaminophen and ibuprofen are the two most popular pain relievers sold without a prescription. They are both sold in generic form. This means that you can buy them under their generic names for a fraction of the price of the name brands.

118

Rubbing alcohol is a dangerous poison. Don't drink it.

119

Sometimes taking lots of baths can cause vaginal yeast infections. If this is a problem, stop taking baths!

120

Don't pick at your pimples or whiteheads. You'll get scars. Use benzoyl peroxide or ask your doctor for Retin-A.

121

There is a new, non-prescription painkiller on the market, called Orudis. It's similar to Aleve (naproxyn). Use it if generic ibuprofen doesn't work well, but it may bother your stomach, so take it with food.

122

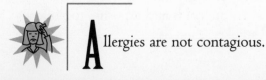

Allergies are not contagious.

123

"Crabs" are little insects that love to live in pubic hairs. They look like tiny whitish specks of dust. They itch! You generally catch them from touching a person or infected bedding. If you get crabs, see your doctor—you need a prescription shampoo.

124

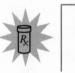

The drugstore pills that help you stay awake just contain caffeine. Have some coffee, it's cheaper.

125

If you are a woman, keep track of when you expect your period. This will help you deal with premenstrual misery, and you'll also know if your period is late.

126

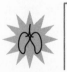

If you have asthma the things that may make you feel worse are colds and exposure to pollen, dust, and smoke.

127

Doctors lead stressful lives and have seen horrible tragedies. If doctors sometimes seem distant and insensitive, this may be why. Just be aware of this, and you'll interact better with your doctor.

128

A cough suppressant keeps you from coughing. The one found in most drugstore cold remedies is called dextromethorphan. It works for mild coughs. If your cough keeps you up at night, see your doctor; you may need a prescription cough medicine.

129

"Flesh-eating disease" is a bacteria that has been around for a long time. It is not a new disease, and it can be treated. If you see signs of infection such as redness, warmth, swelling, or pus, see your doctor right away.

130

You will probably have back pain at some point in your life; most people do. If you are older than fifty, or have numbness and tingling or can't walk, see a neurosurgeon. He will probably order a test called an MRI to make sure that all you have is regular old back pain caused by muscle strain or spasm.

131

Don't open a burn blister. If the blister is opened, it's more likely to get infected.

How should I take care of a cut or scratch?

Clean it well with soap and water or povidone-iodine

Keep it covered and dry

Put antibiotic ointment on it

132

If you have a cold or sinus pressure, use steam treatments. Five times a day boil some water, then cover the bowl and your head with a towel to make a tent. Breathe the steam up through your nose for ten minutes. You'll get better much faster. Don't burn yourself.

133

Women take longer to get sexually aroused than men. This is a fact of life worth remembering.

134

An antihistamine is a cure for allergic reactions. The most common one is called diphenhydramine. This is the generic name; the brand name is Benadryl. Buy the generic! Be aware, however, that most antihistamines will make you sleepy.

135

Ask your dentist how to get in touch with him on weekends, or call some Sunday night and find out if he is reachable during off hours. If you can't reach him or a "covering" dentist, get another dentist!

When should I go to the emergency room with dizziness?

———

Always!

136

If spicy foods bother your stomach, don't eat them. Remember, your body knows best!

137

Stubbed toes often get purple and swollen. Use ice and elevation to get the swelling down. Unless the toe is really deformed, you don't need an X-ray. Take some cotton and put it between your injured toe and one next to it, then gently tape them together. This will support the hurt toe. Wear sneakers until it gets better.

138

Premenstrual syndrome (PMS) can be truly horrible; you are not imagining this.

139

If you are a woman and don't feel like taking your calcium supplement, just watch a hunched over little old lady try to cross the street. That could be you in later years if you don't take your calcium now. Try the orange juice and the bread that are enriched with extra calcium.

140

Burns that blister are a problem if they become infected. Cover all blistered burns carefully and use triple antibacterial ointment to prevent infection. The drugstore brand is fine; the name brands are a waste of money.

141

Some common reasons for nausea are flu, food poisoning, or pregnancy, as well as too much alcohol, caffeine, cigarettes, or stress. If you can't figure out why you are nauseated and fix it, see your doctor.

142

You will live longer if you exercise and eat less fat.

143

The dry air in fall and winter is bad for people with dry, itchy skin. Run a humidifier, use mild soap, bathe as little as possible, and use lotion on your skin.

144

Comparison shop for medicines. Pharmacies often charge different prices for medications, and you can save money by checking around.

145

High blood pressure is a time bomb; it will kill you if it isn't controlled. See your doctor!

146

Poison ivy and poison oak are spread only by touching the plant oil itself. Once you have washed yourself and your clothes with soap and hot water, you can't spread it further. Washing within fifteen minutes of touching the plant is best.

147

You can get poison oak or ivy by touching anything that has the plant oil on it. This includes pet fur, sports equipment, tools, and even shoes. If you can't wash the item, let it sit. The oil will evaporate in three weeks.

148

It seems as if you can spread poison ivy and oak around your body by touching the rash, but you can't. The reason it seems to spread is that the areas that actually touched the plant get red at different times.

149

No one knows how much stress and illness influence each other. It's probably different for each person. Remember, your mind and your body live in the same container, and they have to work together.

150

Half of all injuries to the penis happen during sexual intercourse.

151

Take a decongestant for a runny nose or sinus pain. The most common one is called pseudoephedrine HCL. It has a tendency to keep you awake and may make you feel jumpy. This is the reason drug companies sometimes add antihistamines to cold pills. Antihistamines generally make you sleepy and counteract the jumpiness produced by the decongestant.

152

Antihistamines are good for allergies, but if you just have a cold, don't waste your money on them.

153

Birth control pills are very safe and effective these days, as long as you remember to take them.

154

Nicotine is probably the most addictive drug that you can buy, legally or illegally. People say the nicotine habit is harder to kick than heroin.

155

If taking your medicine bothers your stomach, try eating a piece of chocolate with your pill.

156

If you get chemicals on your hand they can cause bad burns. Lime and bleach can be serious. Run water over the area until your skin feels clean. More is better. If your hand still feels soapy or it stings, keep it under running water until it feels normal. If you have blisters that open, or the burn is painful, see your doctor.

157

Naproxen, which is very similar to ibuprofen, is now sold without a prescription under the brand name Aleve. Currently there is no generic form for sale over-the-counter. Take one, or two at most, three times a day. Some people think it works better than ibuprofen.

158

A cold is caused by a virus, and your body must use its own immune system to get better. Antibiotics will not help! Don't smoke, but do rest, take acetaminophen, and drink lots of fluids. You'll get better, but it may take a week or more.

159

If you have a terrible headache that began when you were exercising, your neck is stiff, and you feel spacey or unusually sleepy, see your doctor right away or go to the emergency room. (See tip 70.)

160

Two percent milk is *high fat*.

161

If it doesn't say "no caffeine" on the label of your soft drink, it probably has some.

162

If you have pain that is located in the right, lower part of your belly and gets steadily worse, go to the emergency room immediately; it could be your appendix.

163

If you have a fever, take two regular strength acetaminophen every four hours. If that doesn't work, you can *also* take two regular strength ibuprofen every six hours. If your fever is higher than 102° F and lasts more than a few days, see your doctor.

164

Remember, your doctor is a person too.

165

Vomiting, like nausea, is a signal that your body is unhappy. Drink plenty of fluids to replace what you are losing.

166

Medicines are always measured in milligrams. There are one thousand milligrams in one gram. This is a common metric measure for weight. You need to know this so you can understand the labels on medicines.

167

Pneumonia is a serious infection in the lungs. You'll almost always get a fever with it, and it's much more common in smokers. If you have a high fever, a cough, and especially if you smoke, see your doctor.

168

If you have acne or even just scattered pimples, try using benzoyl peroxide 10 percent, the ingredient in Clearasil, twice a day. If that doesn't clear them up, see a dermatologist. There are treatments that can really help.

169

Some people feel that they must check things such as the door lock or the stove, or do things in a specific order so they can relax. If you have these feelings and they interfere with your life, see a psychiatrist—she can help.

170

If your ear hurts inside, you may have a middle ear infection. See your doctor.

When should I go to the emergency room with a headache?

If it's the worst headache of your life

If you also have weakness or feel lethargic

If you've had a recent bump on the head

If you've never had headaches before, or if this is a totally different type of headache for you

If you have a high fever or a stiff neck

If you are vomiting so much you can't keep fluids down

171

If your hospital is used for teaching interns and residents, try not to go into the hospital during July and August. These are the months when the young doctors taking care of you are brand new. This could be hazardous to your health.

172

If you have indigestion, both chocolate and mint may worsen your heartburn.

173

If you have liver problems, don't take acetaminophen (Tylenol)—it can further damage your liver.

174

If your headaches are associated with nausea and light hurts your eyes, you may have migraine headaches.

175

Part of the reason alcohol causes a hangover is that it makes you dehydrated. Chase it with water!

176

Colds and flu are usually contagious, but it's hard to know how contagious they are and when they stop being contagious. The safest thing to do is to try to stay away from everyone when you have a cold. Don't use the same glass, do cover your mouth with your elbow when you sneeze, and don't kiss anyone until you feel well again.

177

People often feel depressed after a death in the family or during a loss such as a divorce. If this has happened to you, see a psychotherapist. It's worth it!

178

Drinking extra fluids, and that means drinks without caffeine, will always make you feel better. Just do it!

179

Wear sunglasses with good ultraviolet (UV) protection; they can prevent cataracts and other eye problems when you're older.

What should I do if I have diarrhea?

Drink lots of fluids

Stop eating solids foods until it clears up

Take loperamide if you can't stand it anymore

See your doctor if it lasts more than one week

180

Ankle sprains get better much faster if you prevent the ankle from getting stiff. As soon as possible without hurting it, move your ankle through its full range of motion several times a day. Go to a physical therapist for several sessions if you have the chance. This can prevent sprains in the future.

181

If you are using cough medicine, use it only at night or in the daytime, not both. If you take cough medicine for twenty-four hours every day, it stops working.

182

Diet pills that are sold in drugstores won't help you lose weight. Don't bother buying them.

183

Hives are very common; 20 percent of the population will have them at some point.

184

If your eyes are red, irritated, and have a crusty discharge, it's probably conjunctivitis (an eye infection). This should go away by itself in a few days. If not, see your doctor.

185

Syphilis is a sexually transmitted disease caused by bacteria. It can and must be treated because it can kill you. The first symptom is a painless ulcer, which looks like a hollowed out blister, appearing on your genital area. See your doctor right away; the ulcer will go away, and you might not get other symptoms for months to years.

186

Going bald is a problem for both men and women. Minoxidil works adequately, but hair transplants today are better than they used to be. Don't get depressed; see a skin doctor.

187

If you cut your lip on the outside, and the cut crosses your lip line into regular skin, you must get stitches or it might heal unevenly.

188

If you are traveling in a foreign country—any foreign country—don't drink tap water.

189

A little stress is okay; lots of stress is bad for your health.

190

Throat lozenges and sprays used in moderate amounts are good for painful sore throats.

191

If your skin is dry and itchy in the winter, don't wear wool. Wear cotton clothes and take short, warm showers.

192

If you are raped, here are a few things to remember: Don't change your clothes, don't wash, do call a friend, and immediately call the police and ask for a woman police officer. You must go to the emergency room for an exam. You won't want to, but it will help locate the guilty person. The sooner you do this, the better.

193

Many cities in the United States and Canada have "rape crisis centers" with trained counselors to help. If you are raped, call one.

194

The chance that you will get pregnant from a rape is very small, but there is a pill that will prevent it. You can get it from the emergency room after the exam.

195

If you've sprained your ankle, pick up an Aircast from the pharmacy. (Your medical insurance should pay for it.) Wear it all the time for the first month and then during sports for the six months following your injury.

196

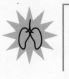

If you have a cold, use decongestants to dry up your runny nose, unless you have prostate or blood pressure problems.

197

Drink lots of water when you travel on an airplane, and get up and walk around every hour. You'll feel better when you get where you're going.

198

If you have the flu, you almost certainly have a virus. See your doctor if you have a high fever for more than a few days, if you have problems breathing, or if you are vomiting so much that you can't keep fluids down.

199

If you eat more fruits and vegetables, you will be less hungry for fatty foods.

200

Never put cotton swabs in your ear canals. Wax is like sweat: it's normal and it comes out by itself. If you smash it back into your ear, you'll end up with a painful wax earplug.

201

Tuberculosis is a bad disease that's spreading again. If you have a persistent cough or notice that you're coughing up blood, especially if you have a fever or wake up sweating at night, see your doctor.

202

If you have ulcers, frequent indigestion, heartburn, or kidney problems, never use ibuprofen or Aleve.

203

Your pharmacist is a great resource. Ask her all the questions you have about medications, especially over-the-counter ones. If necessary she will be happy to call your doctor to clear up any misunderstandings.

204

It's possible to get a rib bruise just from coughing, sneezing, or even laughing a lot.

205

Back pain can be bad, and there's usually not much you can do about it. Ice is the best thing to try first.

206

Crash diets are useless and expensive; don't bother. Save your money and invest in an exercise program.

207

If you are allergic to poison ivy or poison oak, don't eat raw cashews; you might get a nasty rash.

208

If you have lots of earwax, buy some generic liquid carbamide peroxide and a large bulb syringe. Put several drops in your ears and wait thirty minutes. Then use the syringe with warm water to gently wash the wax out. Repeat this routine as needed.

209

Vomiting blood is a bad sign. To make sure the blood came from your stomach and not your nose, blow your nose into a tissue and examine it. If there is no blood on the tissue, the blood probably came from your stomach. See your doctor or go to the emergency room right away.

210

All those expensive sleep aids in the drugstore just contain diphenhydramine, the cheap, generic antihistamine. If you are having trouble sleeping, make sure you aren't drinking caffeine or eating too close to bedtime. If you still can't sleep, then try taking diphenhydramine. Buy the generic; 25–50 milligrams is a good dose.

211

When you get a flu shot, it doesn't protect you from the everyday flu. It only protects you from influenza A and B, nasty flu viruses that cause high fever, chills, and a bad cough.

When should I go to the emergency room with a skin rash?

If you also have trouble breathing

If you have lots of large blisters

If the rash has areas with honey-colored crusting and it hurts

If you also have a headache and fever

212

If you have a cut or a scratch, wash it carefully with soap or diluted povidone–iodine 10 percent. Use an antibiotic ointment on it and cover it with a Band-Aid. It will heal better if it is kept covered and dry.

213

If you find you have little sores in your mouth after having oral sex, stop having oral sex for a week and be more gentle next time. If they don't go away, see your doctor.

214

Most strains and sprains result in damage to the muscles, tendons, or ligaments. You can't see these structures on a regular X-ray.

215

Don't drink and drive.

216

If you suddenly get diarrhea, vomiting, or cramping, you probably have food poisoning. Most of the time it goes away by itself. If you are still sick after two days or have a high fever, blood, or mucus in your stool, see your doctor.

217

If you get your ear pierced and then it gets warm and painful, it's probably infected. Take the earring out, apply hot compresses, and see your doctor right away.

218

Back pain often gets better with rest and ice. Try this first. Do no lifting for one week; this includes groceries, children, and suitcases. Sleep on your side with one pillow between your bent knees. Put ice on your back as often as possible.

219

Fat is a lot worse for you than sugar.

What should I do if I get a bad sunburn?

Use cool compresses on the areas that hurt

Take ibuprofen if it doesn't bother your stomach

If your legs or arms are burned, elevate them

If you get blisters that open up, see your doctor

220

Conjunctivitis, or red eye, is contagious. Don't share washcloths or pillowcases, and wash your hands after touching your eyes.

221

The expensive brand-name liquid cold medicines contain exactly the same ingredients as the cheap generic cold pills.

222

If you have round or oval spots with silvery scales on your elbows or the backs of your legs, you may have a skin disease called psoriasis. See your doctor.

223

If your doctor recommends surgery, you *must* get a second opinion! It's done every day, don't worry about hurting his feelings.

224

Migraine headaches often run in families.

225

If your elbow hurts when you open a door and aches all the time, you may have a type of tendonitis called tennis elbow. Try ice, ibuprofen, gentle exercise, and a special arm band from the drugstore. It can take a long time to go away, sometimes more than a year. If you're really hurting, see an orthopedist.

226

Most nosebleeds are not a big deal. They are caused by dryness in the air, nose blowing or picking, and often by a hot day. Don't worry. If the bleeding won't stop, see your doctor.

227

All the new pain pills that claim to make you sleep better, such as Tylenol PM and Exedrin PM, just contain a mixture of pain medicine and diphenhydramine. If you have pain at night, use a generic pain medicine such as acetaminophen or ibuprofen, and also take 25 milligrams of diphenhydramine. The expensive brand name medicines are a waste of money.

228

Most of the time when you break a bone you can still move it, so don't be fooled. If it really hurts, get an X-ray.

229

If you notice sores on your penis or vaginal area within hours after having sex, you may be allergic to the chemicals in your spermicide. Change your condom brand and don't worry unless it happens frequently.

230

Too much alcohol can kill. If a friend has had so much to drink that he won't respond to you, even if you pinch the inside of his arm hard and yell at him, take him to the nearest emergency room. He could die if you don't.

231

The thyroid is a small gland in your neck that controls loads of important stuff in your body. (See tip 338 and tip 488.)

232

If you've strained your back, try rest and ice. If it still hurts, try massage and stretching. Put a moderate heating pad on your back for five minutes only or take a short warm shower. Then get your spouse or a friend to massage the painful muscles. Follow with some easy stretches, holding the positions for several minutes. Don't bounce! Then ice it for ten minutes. Repeat this process as many times as possible.

233

Canker sores in your mouth hurt! Mix generic diphenhydramine liquid and Kaopectate together one-to-one, swish the mixture around in your mouth, then *spit it out*. Do this four times a day. If it doesn't help, ask your pharmacist for some 2 percent zylocaine (a local anesthetic) and add it to the mixture, or ask him to make the mixture for you.

234

If you have any type of kidney problem, check with your doctor before taking ibuprofen or naproxen.

235

If you have a scaly, itchy rash in just one area, think about it. Do you scratch it all the time? If so, stop! This should fix it.

236

The rule for getting older is, *use it or lose it!* This means if you stop using your brain or your body, you'll settle into stagnant old age. Stay active!

237

If you are using eye drops for conjunctivitis, don't touch the dropper to your eye. If you do, wash it well with soap and water so you don't reinfect yourself.

238

If you are bitten by a snake, don't kill the snake or waste time trying to identify it. Get to a hospital immediately.

239

You don't have to suffer from acne anymore. See your doctor.

240

If you notice small, white, wormlike creatures in your stool, and you have itching around your rectal area, especially at night, you may have pinworms. It's no big deal! Ask your pharmacist for the right medicine: It's called Pyrantel Pamoate. You don't need a prescription.

241

If you use your asthma inhaler more than four times a day, it can be dangerous. Don't do it. If you feel you need more help, see your doctor!

242

If you are taking acetaminophen, always check the amount of drug in the pills. Never take more than 4,000 milligrams in one day. Most people don't need more than 650 milligrams every four to six hours. Do not overuse this drug; it's dangerous!

243

It's tempting to use heat on a pulled muscle because it feels better right away. Don't. Heat will actually make it worse. Use ice instead.

244

Some of the signs of depression are trouble sleeping, change in appetite, decreased energy, and feeling hopeless. If you feel some of these things, see your doctor or a psychiatrist. There are new medicines and treatments that can really make you feel better.

245

Don't panic—foods such as tomatoes, red peppers, and red Jell-O can look like blood in your stool.

246

Never go to the emergency room between four and six in the morning, if you can possibly avoid it. That's when all doctors are at their worst.

247

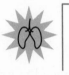

If you cough up blood, make sure it actually came from your lungs and not your nose. Blow your nose and look for blood to make sure. If the blood is definitely coming from your lungs, see your doctor.

248

It turns out that people who eat mostly fruits, vegetables, pasta, and olive oil live a *long time*. Use olive oil instead of butter, and eat more pasta with vegetables.

249

Swollen glands in your neck are usually caused by a minor infection. These glands are part of the lymph system in your body that is responsible for draining away infection. When the glands become swollen, they are doing their job! If you notice sore glands in your neck or under your arms and you feel fine, don't worry! But if they last more than a week or two, see your doctor.

250

If your teeth are sensitive to heat and cold, try the special toothpastes for sensitive teeth. If they still bother you, see your dentist.

251

To get a cut to stop bleeding, apply direct, constant pressure for ten minutes, and elevate it if possible.

252

If you have small red bumps on your shaved legs, it's probably ingrown hairs. Shave less often, scrub hard with a rough skin sponge, and use a lotion with the highest percentage "fruit acids" (alpha hydroxy acids) you can find.

253

The very best time to exercise is whenever you can.

254

Chest pain is worrisome, but if you are younger than thirty-five, you have much less to worry about. Heart attacks in people younger than thirty-five are much less common.

When should I go to the emergency room with an ankle injury?

If you heard a loud pop when you injured it, and you can't extend your toes forward

If you've tried applying ice and elevating it, but you still can't walk on it after two days

If it's so painful you can't sleep

255

If your ears feel stuffed up, and you are planning to fly in a plane, take decongestants the day before and during the flight. On the plane chew gum to help clear your ears.

256

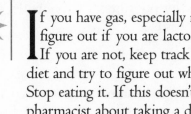

If you have gas, especially if it has a nasty smell, first figure out if you are lactose intolerant. (See tip 101). If you are not, keep track of the vegetables in your diet and try to figure out which one causes the gas. Stop eating it. If this doesn't work, ask your doctor or pharmacist about taking a drug called Flatulex. Take it as directed, but be aware that it may affect your other medications.

257

A boil is a large, painful pimple. Use hot compresses every hour to get the boil to come to a head. You can open it using gentle pressure or a sterilized needle (see tip 40). Drain the pus out, clean it with povidone–iodine, and cover it with antibiotic ointment and a gauze dressing. It may continue to drain for several days, but if the pain and redness are getting better, you can skip the doctor visit. If you have increased pain and redness, see your doctor.

258

Nothing is free. If you take antibiotics, you may get a yeast infection. Antibiotics change normal vaginal bacteria and can cause an overgrowth of yeast.

259

If you have pain in one or both of your testicles that has come on over the course of hours or days, and especially if you can feel a distinct area on the testicle that is sore, see your doctor. Go to the emergency room if the pain began very suddenly.

260

If you normally wear contact lenses and your eyes feel uncomfortable for some reason, take out your contacts and see your eye doctor.

261

If you have a headache, take the strongest pain medicine on your bathroom shelf, drink something with caffeine, and massage the muscles of your head and neck.

What should I do if I have hemorrhoids?

Sit in warm baths whenever you can

Use a cream with pramoxine in it

Take stool softeners or use fiber-based laxatives

262

If your itchy, dry skin starts to get red with honey-colored crusts on it, see your doctor. It's infected.

263

The brand-name cold remedies and pain medicines are the same as the generic. Check the ingredients, and you will usually find they are exactly the same. Don't be intimidated by the long names—check the glossary in the back of this book or ask your pharmacist to explain them to you. (See tip 47.)

264

The usual causes of urinary tract infections in women include forgetting to urinate after sex and wiping back to front instead of the other way.

265

Margarine is probably not good for you. Substitute olive oil whenever you can. If you want real butter, have just a little bit.

266

Rabies is more common than it used to be. Raccoons, skunks, foxes, bats, as well as cats and dogs can carry the virus. Squirrels don't. If you are bitten by one of these animals, you must capture it and take it to a vet. Then go to the emergency room or see your doctor.

267

If you have trouble swallowing pills, try this: To take tablets and solid caplets, fill your mouth with water and tilt your head back so the pill goes down easily. For capsules and gelcaps, which float, after filling your mouth with water, tilt your head forward slightly, then swallow.

268

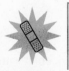

Psychotherapy is good for everyone. Try it!

269

If you are playing sports or running and hear a loud pop then notice that the back of your ankle hurts and it's hard to move your foot, you may have injured your Achilles tendon. See your doctor or go to the emergency room immediately.

270

Make sure you know if your health insurance company pays for medications. Ask the doctor or pharmacist what your medication will cost and find out if there is a generic (less expensive) brand that will work as well.

271

If you have back or neck pain, get your spouse or someone else to massage your back. He should put his hands on your back and rub the muscles as if he were kneading bread dough. This may hurt a little bit, but relaxing, breathing deeply, and working the soreness out of the muscles is crucial. (See tip 232.)

272

There is now a vaccine for chicken pox. If you haven't had chicken pox, get the vaccine!

273

Sun worshipping causes skin cancer. It can kill you.

274

Eating is a bit like shopping. If you try to get the best nutritional value for your calorie, you'll have fewer problems with your weight and probably live longer. For example, plain popcorn is a better bargain than deep-fried cheese.

275

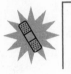

All cuts cause scars.

276

The drugs that claim to be great for your sinuses are just decongestants with added pain medicine. If you have sinus pain, take a generic pain medicine and decongestant. It's cheaper.

277

If you get a speck in your eye, try to wash it out with plenty of water. If you can't, see an eye doctor or go to the emergency room.

278

If you get food poisoning, drink as much clear fluid as possible, stop eating, and rest. Take generic Kaopectate if the diarrhea is really bothering you. After you begin to feel better, start eating slowly. Toast, noodle soups, bananas, and Jell-O are good things to start with. Add milk products and vegetables to your diet last.

279

If sex isn't fun for you, find out why. Buy a book or videotape that explains how to have better sex. Don't be embarrassed; after all, your body didn't come with instructions.

280

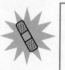

Even for weekend athletes, frequent ankle sprains are a problem because the ligaments holding the ankle together loosen, and the joint becomes slightly unstable. This can often be improved by physical therapy. Ask your doctor to prescribe some therapy if your ankles are weak.

281

Sometimes your doctor is cranky because she's just tired. She might have been up all night, had a patient die, or maybe she has problems at home. Ignore your doctor's mood and get the care you need.

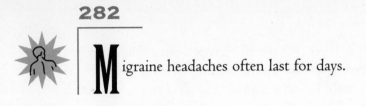

282

Migraine headaches often last for days.

283

If you hurt your nose and it looks really crooked, see your doctor to document the injury. If you need to have your nose straightened after an injury, your insurance company may refuse to pay for it. They'll say that they don't pay for cosmetic surgery, and without proof of an injury, your nose may end up crooked forever.

284

Too much caffeine can make heart skips, called PVCs, worse. (See tip 66.) If they are bothering you, cut down your caffeine and see your doctor.

285

If you notice your heart skipping, cough immediately. This should help it to stop skipping.

When should I go to the emergency room with chest pain?

If it feels like someone is sitting on your chest

If you also have shortness of breath, sweating, or nausea

If the pain is severe

If you've been using cocaine

If you are also having any problems breathing

286

Shingles is actually the chicken pox virus that has returned to irritate you. It usually hurts even before you get a rash. If you get a rash like chicken pox in a small area, especially if it hurts, see your doctor right away.

287

AIDS will kill you. If you are having sex and don't want to die, protect yourself with a condom.

288

If you need stitches, see your doctor or go to the emergency room right away! The longer you wait, the greater the chances that you will get an infection.

289

Many women have trouble having orgasms, and only a small percentage actually have orgasms during intercourse without clitoral stimulation. If you are a woman and your partner doesn't understand this, tell him!

290

For back pain, take three or four ibuprofen three times a day with food, or two extra strength acetaminophen three times a day. The ibuprofen is probably better if your stomach can take it. If this doesn't work, substitute two Aleve for the ibuprofen.

291

Alcohol is a dangerous drug. With long-term overuse, it causes liver disease, heart problems, and death.

292

If your jaw hurts when you open it very wide, you may have a joint problem called TMJ. It's like a sprained ankle in your jaw. Don't eat chewy foods; do use ice and rest your jaw.

293

If you have high blood pressure, diabetes, or thyroid problems, do not take decongestants of any kind.

294

Broken toes are not usually set; they heal themselves. But they hurt a lot!

When should I go to the emergency room with abdominal pain?

If there is any chance that you are pregnant

If you can't drink fluids or eat

If you also have urinary discomfort or vaginal discharge

If you are vomiting blood or bleeding from your rectum

If the pain began very suddenly and is severe

If the pain is constant and getting worse

295

Hives look like a big, flat, red, itchy rash that seems to move around. They are usually caused by an allergic reaction to something. Figure out what you are allergic to and stop it. Use diphenhydramine pills and cool compresses. The hives will probably go away on their own.

296

If your doctor has prescribed an asthma inhaler, make sure your pharmacist shows you exactly how to use it.

297

If you get an insect in your ear, pour some mineral oil in your ear canal. This will kill the bug. Have a friend take it out or see your doctor.

298

If you feel as if you are getting a urinary tract infection, try drinking lots of cranberry juice to see if it clears up by itself. It probably won't; see your doctor.

299

There are doctors who specialize in geriatrics, the care of the elderly. If you are older than seventy, consider looking for one of these specialists.

300

If you get a painful scratch on your eyeball and you haven't had a tetanus shot in the last five years, you need one. See your doctor.

301

An MRI scan shows most of the things we cannot see on regular x-rays such as tendons, ligaments, cartilage, and discs.

302

If you have trouble sleeping because you keep thinking of more things you have to do, make a list, keep it by your bed, and add to it when you think of something new.

303

Birth control pills do not cause cancer. They probably protect against certain types of cancer.

304

An expectorant medicine makes it easier for the mucus clogging your head and chest to get out. The most common one is guaifenesin. It works well as long as you are drinking plenty of fluids.

305

Be suspicious of all health insurance companies, including HMOs. They are all trying to make a profit. Your good health and welfare are not always their first priority. Carefully check the coverage they are offering and then check out the competition. HMOs often have limitations on which doctor you can see and which hospitals you can go to. They also have disguised caps on how many health care dollars you can spend. Find out about their system for approving a surgery or a procedure. Often if they don't think the surgery is necessary, no matter what your doctors think, they won't pay for it.

306

If your cough won't let up, try holding an ice cube in your mouth until it melts. If this works, do it as often as necessary.

307

Where's the fat? You've got to know. Read the labels on food packages to stay healthy.

308

If you have pain that is located in the right upper part of your belly, it comes and goes, and is clearly worse after eating fatty foods, it may be your gall bladder. Try cutting out all fatty foods and see if that helps. This is not an emergency unless you have a fever or are vomiting so much you can't keep fluids down.

309

If you find that your ears get sore or itchy after swimming, mix 1 pint of rubbing alcohol with five table-spoons of white vinegar and rinse your ear canal with a small amount of this after swimming. This will help dry the canal. Try to keep your ears dry for two weeks—use ear plugs in the shower and avoid swimming. See your doctor if they keep hurting.

310

If you need to see a doctor, try to do it before five P.M.

311

If you break your penis, you'll know. It can happen only when the penis is erect. It can be repaired.

312

If the muscle under your shoulder blade hurts, you're not alone. It's very common. Try ice, ibuprofen, and resting the muscle. This means you should not lift anything with that arm. If it doesn't improve, see your doctor first. If he can't help, so see a chiropractor.

313

Talcum powder is actually bad for rashes and itching. Don't use it!

314

If you have a burn that covers a large area, especially on your hands or face, go to the emergency room or see your doctor immediately.

315

All medical procedures involve some risk.

316

Whitish spots on your throat mean you have an infection. This infection may be caused by a virus and can't be treated with antibiotics. Your doctor will do a throat culture to check for strep, which is a *bacteria* and can be treated.

317

Burns leave scars that can become worse if the burn gets infected.

318

Don't bother trying to lose weight with big time sweating: Your kidneys are smarter than that. You'll just get thirsty and end up having to drink the fluid you lost by sweating. The only way to lose "water weight" is to eat less salt.

319

Cigarettes and excessive alcohol are probably the most harmful and dangerous drugs available.

320

If the skin on your buttocks and the backs of your upper arms is bumpy, don't worry, it's a common problem. Use a lotion with a high percentage of fruit acids. If it still bothers you, see a skin doctor.

321

Do not get tested for AIDS (the HIV virus) at a clinic that requires your name. The result could get into your medical record and keep you from getting insurance in the future. Get tested at an anonymous center where they give you a number and don't require your name. Call an AIDS hotline to find out where to go.

322

A hernia is a piece of gut that sometimes bulges out through a hole in your abdominal wall or groin. It usually goes back in by itself. If it's stuck, it will hurt. See your doctor or go to the emergency room.

323

If you are younger than thirty-five and have a cough and chest pain *when* you take deep breaths, you probably have bronchitis. It is usually caused by a virus. If it lasts more that two weeks, if you have a fever, or if you feel short of breath, see your doctor.

324

If you have dry skin, take short showers with warm water and apply a moisturizer as soon as you get out.

325

Use a body soap such as Dove that doesn't dry out your skin. Ivory and all the deodorant soaps are very drying.

326

Find the number for your local Poison Control center and post it by the phone. Call immediately if someone swallows something harmful.

327

Talk during sex. Tell your partner what you want, what you think about, what you feel.

When should I go to the emergency room with back pain?

If you also have chest pain

If you also have numbness, especially around your tailbone

If you have weakness in your other muscles

If you can't control your bowels or bladder

If you've just had a bad injury or accident

If you also feel dizzy and weak

328

Migraine headaches are terrible, so see your doctor—there is a great new drug called Imitrex.

329

If you have a dark black bowel movement that looks like tar, this means there's blood in it. See your doctor right away, unless you've been using Pepto Bismol. This stuff can make your stool black like tar.

330

If you have a headache all the time, make sure your eyes or teeth are not the source of the problem. Also make sure you are not taking acetaminophen (Tylenol) every day; this can cause a constant rebound headache.

331

One of the easiest birth control methods for women is a drug called Depro Provera. It's very safe, and you get an injection once every three months; that's all.

332

If you have diarrhea it's probably best not to treat it with medicine unless it's really bothering you. If you decide to treat it, use generic loperamide or Kaopectate from the drugstore. Make sure to drink gallons of fluids and see your doctor if it lasts more than one week.

333

If you close your finger in a car door, use ice and elevation to treat it. It's usually not broken, but it's a good idea to see your doctor for an X-ray.

334

If you suspect a skin infection, soak it. Use hot water, but don't burn yourself; throw in some povidone–iodine; and soak the infected area at least five times a day. More is better. If the infected area can't be dunked into the water, hold hot cloths on it. If it's not better in twenty-four hours, see your doctor.

335

Here's a basic rule of responsible health care: Don't order a test unless you plan to change the treatment of the problem based on the results of the test. (See tip 34.)

How often do I need a tetanus shot?

Every ten years if you don't have a new cut or burn

Every five years if you do have a recent cut or burn

336

If you are bitten by a dog, wash the bite carefully and cover it. Make sure the dog has had a rabies shot. If the bite isn't on your face and doesn't need stitches, it's possible you can skip a doctor visit. Watch it carefully for signs of infection: redness, warmth, tenderness, and swelling. If it is healing without these signs, don't worry.

337

Sexually transmitted diseases are one of the leading causes of infertility for women. Protect yourself with a condom.

338

Do you have trouble losing weight, feel tired and cold all the time, and does your skin seems very dry? See your doctor, you may have an underactive thyroid.

339

Preparation H is an outdated remedy containing shark oil. Most doctors do not recommend it.

340

If you have a red, painful place on your eyelid that looks like a pimple, you probably have a sty. Instead of using messy wet hot compresses, hard boil an egg and without removing it from the shell, and without burning yourself, hold it to your eyelid. Keep it there for about ten minutes. Reuse the egg and do this four times a day. If the sty is not gone in two days, see an eye doctor.

341

If you wake up with a stiff neck, put some mild heat on it for ten minutes, massage it, and slowly stretch it out. (This is one of the only times you should use heat.) The pain should go away in one or two days.

342

If you don't want to have sex because you are ashamed of how your body looks, turn off the lights. It's not worth giving up sex just because you want to lose some weight.

343

Asthma kills more people than it once did, and we're not sure why.

344

Having to watch what you eat is a never-ending battle.

345

Ibuprofen, the ingredient in Advil, Motrin, and Nuprin is a great drug for sprains and bruises—unless you have stomach problems.

346

If your ear hurts when you pull on your ear lobe or it feels sore in the canal, you probably have an infection of the ear canal. Keep it dry! If it doesn't go away in a day or so, see your doctor. If you are diabetic, see your doctor immediately! (See tip 309.)

347

If your heel hurts and you have not injured it, you may have ordinary heel pain. Wear sneakers with lots of heel support and elevate and ice your foot whenever possible. Use ibuprofen or acetaminophen and try not to stand or walk too much. If it doesn't go away, see a podiatrist.

348

All good doctors have "on-call coverage." This means that at night and on weekends, one doctor is picked to take care of all the patients in the physicians' group. If you need your doctor during off hours, ask to speak to the "covering doctor." This person will take care of you until your regular doctor can take over. If your doctor doesn't have "on call coverage," get another doctor!

349

Cooperate with your body: it's the only one you have.

350

Heavy lifting can sometimes create what's called a hernia by pushing the gut through a weak place in the abdominal wall. (See tip 322.)

351

If you get your ears pierced make sure the needle is clean and disposable. Rotate the earrings twice a day only and wash your hands before you do.

352

If you touch some poison ivy or oak, buy Burrow's solution from your pharmacy. Mix it as directed and soak some gauze in it. Lay the gauze compresses over the blisters for thirty minutes every three hours. This will make the blisters dry up and go away.

353

If you get poison ivy or oak, short cool tub baths with Aveeno will help the itch. Ask your pharmacist for it.

354

If you *abruptly, suddenly* get pain in your testicles, go to the emergency room immediately! If the pain is from a twisted spermatic cord, you may have only four hours before you *lose* that testicle. Tell the first nurse you see that you are worried about "testicular torsion." This should get her attention.

355

Tetanus is a disease that causes lockjaw. If your last tetanus shot was more than five years ago and you get a cut or burn, you need a tetanus shot. No matter what, you need a booster every ten years.

356

Anxiety is an edgy, nervous, restless feeling that interferes with your daily life. It's awful! If you have this, see a psychotherapist. There are treatments that can help.

357

Don't pick at your skin, you'll get scars and infections.

358

The more you drink, the better your body becomes at processing alcohol. This is not a reason to get drunk.

359

Bee and wasp stings are uncomfortable but not dangerous for most people. They will usually get more swollen and itchy over the first few days. If you have a whole body rash or any trouble breathing go to the emergency room immediately.

360

If you often have pain in your belly and no one knows what to do, you probably have irritable bowel syndrome. It's very common. Many patients with this problem have had many tests or operations that didn't help. Try eating a high fiber diet and avoiding the foods that seem to make your pain worse. Ask your doctor to look at the latest research related to this disease.

361

If your throat is so sore that it hurts too much to swallow food, don't! Just drink things such as juice and chicken broth. Your body will manage fine on liquids for a few days.

362

There is a technique called "ice massage" that can really help pain, especially sore muscles and backs. Fill styrofoam cups with water, and freeze them. Tear off the top part of the cup to use the ice. Rub it lightly back and forth over the sore area in a circular motion. You will first feel coldness, then burning, then aching, then numbness. It won't stop hurting until it gets numb. Do this for ten minutes, no more. After several treatments, you'll find the area feels much better. Try this whenever you have pain. Be careful not to leave the ice on so long that your skin gets white or mottled.

363

There is really no good treatment for a broken rib, except pain control. If you think you might have a broken rib, it will hurt, but don't worry. Use non-prescription painkillers and ice the painful area. If you feel short of breath, go to the emergency room.

364

If you get a scratch on your eyeball it will hurt like crazy! Keep your eye closed with tape and see an eye doctor right away or go to the emergency room. Take whatever pain medicine you have in the house before you go. If you haven't had a tetanus shot within five years, you need one.

365

If you've already gone through menopause and have vaginal bleeding, go to your doctor immediately! Never ignore this type of bleeding, not even for a day!

366

Some drugstore medicines for itch contain lido-caine, a local anesthetic. This doesn't work; use hydrocortisone cream instead.

89

When should I go to the emergency room with a burn?

If it is on your hand or face and has blisters

If it is getting red, warm, and tender and has pus oozing from it

If it was associated with an explosion or smoke inhalation

If it extends over a large area of skin

If it's on your genitals

367

No one really knows what vitamins you should take for great health. It's probably a good idea to take vitamins C and E as well as beta carotene. You can get these in one pill, often called an antioxidant formula. Don't forget to eat plenty of fruits and vegetables.

368

Doctors often do unnecessary tests to protect themselves. Don't be afraid to ask your doctor *why* she has ordered a test on you.

369

Learn to dance, play the piano, read new books, travel; strive to stay young.

370

If you bite your fingernails and cuticles, you are more likely to get an infection under the fingernail.

371

Spraining your knee is a particularly difficult problem because it's a complex joint and you depend on it constantly. If you hurt your knee, use ice, elevation, a tight brace that keeps your knee from moving, and crutches for one week. If it still hurts after one to two weeks of *total* rest—no cheating!—see an orthopedic specialist.

372

Dandruff can usually be controlled by using dandruff shampoos. If you are using these and your scalp is still flaky, see a skin specialist.

373

If you've met someone you want to continue having sex with, keep using condoms for six months. At that point, if you've both been faithful to each other, you should both have blood tests for AIDS. If they are negative, it's probably okay to stop using condoms. Have another test after one year.

374

A groin pull is a deep, painful muscle strain that often takes a long time to heal. It will hurt when you walk or go up stairs. Use ice and ibuprofen and rest it for several weeks.

What should I do with a painful ingrown toenail?

Soak it in hot water as often as possible

Elevate the toe

Cut out a wedge-shaped piece, including the cuticle, on the painful side

See a podiatrist

375

Aches and pains that keep you awake, or wake you up from sleep, are usually more significant than ones that don't.

376

Smoking is probably the single worst thing you can do to your health.

377

Don't drink apple juice when you have diarrhea.

378

If your ear hurts, you've been treated with antibiotics twice, and especially if you smoke, see an ear specialist, right away.

379

Doctors rarely take out tonsils these days. Tonsils are part of the immune system, but we don't know exactly what they do. Unless they bother you more than five times a year, it's safer to leave them in.

380

Tension headaches usually begin with stress and are sometimes relieved by ice packs, massage, and gentle stretching of the neck muscles.

381

If you have open sores on your genitals, this increases your chances of getting AIDS if you have unprotected sex. So don't.

382

If you get a chemical in your eye, rinse the eye with water for ten minutes, making sure to turn your head so the chemical stays out of your uninjured eye, then go to the emergency room as fast as possible. Tell the registration person that you have a chemical burn to the eye and that if you have to wait to see a doctor you must have somewhere to wash your eye. Keep running water over your eye until you see a doctor.

383

If your face, head, and teeth hurt; you have a runny nose; and the pain increases when you bend over, it's probably your sinuses. Use steam treatments (See tip 132) and visit your doctor.

384

If you get round or oval patches of whitish or reddish skin on your upper trunk that don't itch, see a skin doctor. You may have a fungus.

385

If you fall and hurt your hip, especially if it really hurts when you walk, see your doctor. If you are older than sixty, make sure you get an X-ray.

386

The most important thing you can do to make an emergency room visit better and faster is to know your health history. More than 50 percent of the work during an emergency room visit is simply obtaining that information. Write down your medications, medical problems, procedures and surgeries, and their results, with dates, on an index card. Keep this card in your wallet; you will receive better and faster medical care.

387

Nothing is free. Even if your health insurance company pays your bills today, someday someone else will pay that bill. The odds are that that someone will be you the next time your insurance rates rise.

388

Watch your fat intake by using nonfat dairy products, skipping snack foods, and eating less meat.

389

Get into a routine before you go to sleep. Putting on pajamas, reading, or just sitting in a special chair will remind your body that it's time to sleep.

390

Back and neck pain are often helped by chiropractic treatment, massage therapy, or acupuncture. One or all of these will help most people. Try them; it's impossible to predict which one will help you. Make sure the person you see has been to a respectable school and has been well trained.

391

If you have constant pain in your shoulder, elbow, or wrist, you may have tendonitis. Try ice and ibuprofen then see your doctor or an othopedic specialist.

392

Everyone is different. For some people a sprained ankle is torture, for others a broken arm is no big deal.

393

If your throat hurts so much that you really can't swallow, see your doctor or go to the emergency room right away.

394

If you have a whitish discharge like cottage cheese coming from your vagina, accompanied by itching and burning, you probably have a yeast infection. Use the cream you can buy in the drugstore. If this doesn't help, ask your doctor about a new drug called Diflucan that cures this problem with just one pill.

395

If you suddenly feel that the room is spinning around, especially after abrupt head movements such as sitting up in bed, you probably have vertigo. If you are generally well, don't worry! Try to tolerate it for a while and it will probably go away. If you have any other symptoms such as hearing loss, or if it lasts more than a few days, see your doctor.

396

Dizziness is different than vertigo. Dizziness is more like feeling light-headed or like you might pass out. The most common cause is not drinking enough fluids. If you find that you are dizzy when you stand up suddenly, drink lots of fluids. If the dizziness lasts, see your doctor.

397

If you are dizzy and it feels as if everything is starting to go black, or if you sometimes have areas of blackness at the edges of your vision, see your doctor. These could be signs of a stroke.

398

There really is a hole in the ozone, and it really is causing more skin cancer, especially the type that can kill you. Wear sunscreen and a hat.

399

Do you want to live longer? Wear your seatbelt!

When should I go to the emergency room with a cough?

If you have a fever higher than 102 degrees and feel very ill

If you can't stop coughing and can't sleep

If you feel short of breath and can't get enough air

If you are coughing up blood

If you've inhaled food or a foreign object

If you've just inhaled smoke or chemicals

400

Before taking extra iron, ask your doctor—it may not be good for you.

401

If you are a man and it hurts when you urinate, you have to go all the time, and you have an achy pain in your lower back area, you may have prostatitis. See your doctor; go especially quickly if you also have fever and chills.

402

If you get a rash under your arms, it may be from a new deodorant.

403

If you fall onto your back or have an accident and then notice some blood in your urine, see your doctor or go to the emergency room.

404

Groundskeepers use lime to paint lines on baseball diamonds and football fields. If you get this on your skin it can cause a bad burn. Run water over it and see your doctor if it continues to hurt.

405

Every time you get behind the wheel after having *even one drink,* you are risking your life.

406

If you call your doctor and the secretary tells you that he is on vacation or gone for the day, ask to talk with the *on-call* or *covering* doctor. If you are told that doctor is unavailable right now, ask when you will be called back. Be persistent! If you don't hear from the doctor within two hours, call back.

407

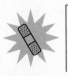

Alcohol is lousy for cleaning a cut; it doesn't kill germs very well. Use povidone–iodine instead.

What should I do if my neck always hurts?

Ice it

Have someone massage it

Lower your stress level

See a chiropractor or your doctor

408

If you are a woman on a diet, sometimes you may feel shaky and weak, especially during exercise. This is probably not low blood sugar, but may happen because you need more protein. Try eating more protein, especially before you exercise.

409

Don't use heat on sprains!

410

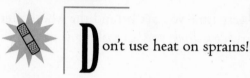

If you have genital herpes and it hurts like crazy when you urinate, buy some zinc oxide from the drugstore and cover the painful lesions. This will lessen the pain when you urinate.

411

If you swallow something you shouldn't, such as a tooth or a fish bone, and it doesn't hurt, don't worry.

412

Chiropractors can help back pain. Traditional Western medicine doesn't really understand how the treatment works, but it does, for some people. Make sure you really need all the X-rays chiropractors order and insist they also be read by a licensed radiologist who is an M.D.

413

If you hurt your nose, it will probably swell and bruise. Put ice on it right away, keep your head elevated, don't blow your nose, and stop the bleeding. Broken noses are not set; they usually mend themselves. (See tip 281.)

414

If you feel stressed, take a meditation class of some kind. It will teach you ways to handle your stress.

415

Hemorrhoids are just enlarged veins that poke out and hurt. They usually get more painful when you pass stool.

416

Women must have a PAP smear once a year. This test screens for cancer of the cervix. Don't worry: It doesn't hurt.

417

The best way to sleep is on your side, with a pillow tucked between your bent knees.

418

You need stitches if your cut is large, over a joint, on your hand, or if it pulls apart by itself.

419

If you suddenly develop an itchy rash, ask yourself if you have used any new products such as detergent, lotion, fabric softener, or shampoo. If so, stop using the product and see if the rash goes away. This could take one to ten days. Use diphenhydramine pills, the ingredient in Benadryl, and 1 percent hydrocortisone cream for the itch. If most of the rash is on your face, hands, or groin, see your doctor.

420

The problem with things such as chronic back pain and arthritis is that we can't do much about them. If you have been told by a doctor that your pain is not caused by a serious disease, and you've had a second opinion, try to ignore the pain.

421

Emergency department care costs about three times what medical care costs in a doctor's office. Everybody ends up paying for this. Try to see your regular doctor—it's worth it.

422

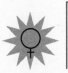

If you are prone to PMS, watch your caffeine and salt intake, use ibuprofen for headaches, and rest. Just assume you'll feel vulnerable and crummy for a few days and don't forget to warn your friends.

423

If you mix cement for a home project be very careful: You can get terrible burns. Don't let it touch your hands or knees. If you get cement on yourself, wash with water for one hour and see your doctor.

424

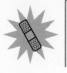

If your forearm and last two fingers feel numb and tingly it's probably your ulnar nerve, also known as the "funny bone." Make sure you are not putting pressure on it when you drive, work, or sleep, and it should go away.

425

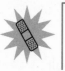

If your throat is so sore and swollen that it interferes with your breathing, go to the emergency room immediately!

426

Rib bruises are very painful. You will have pain every time you breath or move; they hurt all the time. Expect them to get worse for the first week or more, but after that the pain should slowly start to get better.

427

If your primary care doctor suggests that you take a psychiatric medication such as an antidepressant, ask to be referred to a psychiatrist. There are so many new drugs on the market it's almost impossible for a general practitioner to know all about them. These drugs can really do wonderful things for your life if correctly prescribed.

Ringworm, jock itch, and athlete's foot are all caused by the same fungus, which likes warm, wet, dark places. If you have it, dry the area with a cool hair dryer carefully after bathing. Try one of the drugstore creams or use a spray, but don't use anything with talc in it. Read the labels. If you still have itching and scaling, see your doctor.

429

If you have a dental emergency and can't reach a dentist, call the nearest hospital associated with a teaching center. They will probably have an emergency dental clinic.

430

If you have chest pain that feels like someone is sitting on your chest, go to the emergency room *immediately.*

431

If you are using eye drops for conjunctivitis, apply them every two hours. Put them in your uninfected eye every other time.

432

 Don't eat ordinary airplane food. It generally tastes bad and is loaded with fat. Always order a special lowfat or vegetarian meal. If you forget to order one twenty-four hours in advance, pack a lunch.

433

 Diarrhea is sometimes caused by nerves. It usually vanishes with your stress.

434

 Most of the drugstore medicines for fungal infections are generic clotrimazole or miconazole. They all work pretty well. If you don't get better after using one, see your doctor.

435

 Make sure you know what your health insurance company requires before you go to an emergency room. Sometimes if you don't get preapproval from your primary care doctor, the company won't pay for the visit.

436

If you have hives and difficulty breathing, go to the emergency room or call an ambulance.

437

There is some evidence that vitamin E is good for preventing heart attacks.

438

If the area around your fingernail gets red and painful, soak it in hot water mixed with povidone–iodine. If this doesn't help, keep soaking it until you can see yellowish pus under the skin. Then see your doctor; it needs to be opened. If it opens by itself, gently press the pus out, apply antibiotic ointment, and keep it covered. This can also happen to your toenail, but it's less likely.

439

Shoulder injuries are painful, but they often get better with ice and a sling. If you are using a sling, make sure to take it off several times a day and walk your fingers up a wall so that your shoulder doesn't get stiff. If you are older than fifty, make sure you do this! If the pain is terrible, see your doctor.

When should I go to the emergency room with an eye problem?

If you have suddenly lost your vision

If you have something in your eye

If your vision is abnormal, especially in only one eye

440

If you cut yourself badly late at night and wait until the next morning to see the doctor, it will probably be too late for stitches.

441

If you need stitches and don't get them right away, there's a good chance that your cut will take a long time to heal.

442

If you have a fever and pain in your back along with the signs of a urinary tract infection, see your doctor right away; you could have a kidney infection. If you are also vomiting and have a fever, go to the emergency room.

443

If ibuprofen doesn't help your pain, use Naproxyn, the ingredient in the brand name pill Aleve. Don't use it if you have ulcers or other stomach problems.

444

Today's street drugs are more dangerous than ever.

445

If you notice a rash where your belt buckle touches, you may be allergic to the metal in the buckle. Take it off.

446

Bruised fingers hurt! Elevate them as much as possible—most of the pain comes from the swelling. Cover them with a bulky dressing to keep from hitting them again.

447

If you have diarrhea, always drink plenty of fluids to make up for what you are losing.

448

If your voice is hoarse and this persists after you've had two courses of antibiotics, see a throat specialist immediately! If you smoke, this is even more important.

449

Natural isn't always good. Cyanide is natural but it still kills you.

What should I do if my sinuses are stuffed up?

Put your head over a pot of boiling water, cover it with a towel, and breathe the steam five times a day for five to ten minutes

Take the generic form of Sudafed

Do not use the sprays that claim to clear up your nose—they are addictive

Drink plenty of fluids and if you don't get better in a week, see your doctor

450

The only birth control method that protects you against AIDS and other diseases is a condom.

451

If you don't stitch a cut on your face you are more likely to get a noticeable scar. If the cut is in a very visible place, try to find a plastic surgeon. Otherwise see your doctor or go to the emergency room.

452

If you get stitches on your face, they should be removed after four or five days. If the doctor tells you to come back in a week, ask why. If he doesn't give you a good reason, come back in five days.

453

The treatment for acute pain from an injury differs from the treatment for long-term pain such as from arthritis. (See tip 420 and tip 474.)

Health food stores sell many kinds of dietary supplements such as protein powders and pills that claim to reduce fat. Keep in mind that these products are not tested or approved by the FDA (Federal Drug Administration) and may be dangerous. Standard multivitamins and antioxidant combinations are generally considered safe.

Head lice are tiny insects that look like little white specks and live on the scalp. Try a remedy from the drugstore but remember to treat everyone in the house. You must wash all the sheets and towels in very hot water and use a hot dryer. Everything may need a second treatment. If the bugs don't go away, see your doctor.

If you are a woman, you release an egg once a month, approximately two weeks after your period starts. This is the time you are most likely to get pregnant. Sometimes when that egg comes out it's a little painful. If it's very painful, and the pain lasts more than four hours, see your doctor.

457

Car accidents are no fun. If you've been in a minor car accident, expect to feel sore for one to five days after the accident. Your shoulders, neck, and back will probably hurt and get worse during the first few days. Take ibuprofen three times a day, ice all the areas that hurt, take it easy, and stay home if possible. Your body has had a shock, and it will take time to recover. If your neck really hurts over the bony places in the back, see your doctor.

458

Children die every day because they don't wear helmets. Don't let your kid out the door to bike, skateboard, or skate without one!

459

The ticks that cause Lyme disease are tiny—much, much smaller than the ticks you find on your dog.

460

If you are younger than thirty-five, have sharp chest pain when you breath deeply, and can duplicate your pain by pushing on the front of your chest, you probably have an irritation of the chest wall. Try taking ibuprofen. If it lasts more than two weeks, see your doctor.

461

If you are bitten by a snake, don't make a cut and try to suck the venom out. It doesn't work. Take a wide band, like a handkerchief, and wrap it tightly around the limb just an inch above the bite. Put a splint on the limb and try to keep it at heart level. Don't bother with ice or anything else. Get to a hospital immediately.

462

If you have extremely bad pain that goes from your lower back around into your groin, you may have a kidney stone. Drink as much liquid as possible. See your doctor or go to the emergency room.

463

If you have bright red blood in your stool, check to see if it's from hemorrhoids. Use a hand mirror. Hemorrhoids look like swollen purple grapes. If hemorrhoids are the problem, take frequent warm baths, and use a stool softener and a generic ointment (not a cream) with pramoxine in it.

464

If you cut yourself and get blood on your clothes, pour hydrogen peroxide directly on the spot and rub until the blood comes out. Then wash the clothing.

465

If you are stung by an insect and have lots of redness, swelling, and itching you should use ice packs, elevate the bite if possible, and use diphenhydramine pills and 1 percent hydrocortisone cream. Go to the doctor if you have problems breathing.

466

If you are stung by an insect on the hand or the face, expect it to get very swollen. Don't worry, it will go away. (See tip 465.)

467

If you notice sores on your genitals, and they last more than a few days, you may have some type of sexually transmitted disease. See your doctor.

468

Acupuncture is an ancient Chinese medical treatment which has been used for thousands of years. Western researchers have shown that it raises the level of natural pain relievers in the body. It probably also works in ways we don't understand. Make sure your acupuncturist uses new disposable needles. Don't worry, the needles don't hurt!

469

If you switch to lowfat foods such as fruit, vegetables, and bread, you'll lose weight more easily.

470

If you hit your head, and you are unconscious for any length of time, have someone drive you to the emergency room.

471

If you hit your head, the worst thing that could happen is bleeding in the brain. It's hard to tell when people have bleeding, and the only way to find out is by doing a CAT scan, an expensive test. After any head injury, have someone watch you carefully for repeated vomiting, extreme sleepiness, severe headache, and balance problems. Have someone wake you up in the middle of the night; if you can't be woken, an ambulance should be called right away!

472

In the vagina, lots of bacteria live happily together—this is normal. Sometimes their cheerful balance becomes upset by stress—a bubble bath, an antibiotic—and sometimes it happens for no particular reason. When this happens, you may get itching, a discharge, or an irritated feeling. Try to stop whatever is upsetting the balance and see your doctor.

473

Tetanus lives in dirt and dust. It's dangerous; don't ignore it. Get a tetanus shot. (See tip 355.)

474

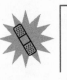

There are specialty pain control centers for people with long-term, chronic pain. Check the phone book for a pain clinic; they are usually attached to a teaching hospital. These places really work!

475

If you have a mole and it looks darker than it did previously, is more uneven, or is bigger than a pencil eraser, see your doctor.

476

 Sometimes having diarrhea or hemorrhoids can cause small sores around your rectal area. Clean them gently and use an antibiotic ointment.

477

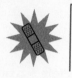 A cast is meant to keep your broken limb still. Most of the time you can use the limb if you try. Don't! If it's broken, *don't use it at all.* If you do, it may not heal.

478

 Ingrown toenails are not fun. If you tend to get them, buy a special toenail clipper with a straight edge on it. About once a month, soak your feet in warm soapy water and immediately afterward clip your toenails. Cut close to the edge, directly down the side toward the base of the toe nail as far as you can go without hurting yourself. Then take the sliver in your fingers and gradually pull it out, taking as much of the cuticle with you as possible. Gently scrape out any part of the nail that didn't come out with the sliver, including the soft cuticle than builds up at the side of the nail. Then dab some antibiotic ointment on your toenail. This routine should prevent ingrown nails. If it doesn't work, see a podiatrist.

When should I go to the emergency room with an allergic reaction?

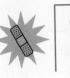

479

If your ingrown toenail has started to hurt or get red, it's probably infected. Soak it in hot water with some povidone—iodine in it. This may cure the infection and allow you to remove the ingrown part (See tip 478.) If it's still red and painful, see a podiatrist.

If you have any trouble breathing (call an ambulance)

If your throat feels tight

If you have severe vomiting

If you have a history of severe allergic reactions

480

Always buckle your seat belt before starting the car. Buy a car with an airbag if possible.

481

A scab is nature's answer to a Band-Aid. Leave it alone!

482

Some people think vitamin C stops colds. No one has proven this, but it probably won't hurt unless you take more than 3 grams a day.

483

Sitting in the sun causes wrinkles and makes you look much older than you really are. If you want a tan, try self-tanning lotions: They look great and don't cause cancer and wrinkles like the sun does.

484

If you want to buy the antihistamine diphenhydramine in a generic form, check the sleep aid section of your drugstore. It may be cheaper to buy it packaged as a sleep aid. Check the dosage and the amount of pills in the bottle.

485

If you are still menstruating, you can get pregnant any time you have intercourse without using birth control. It doesn't matter if it's one time only, if you have your period, or if you've never been pregnant. Always use birth control unless you are positive that you want a baby.

486

If you get something in your eye that won't come out, rinse it with water for an hour. If it still won't come out, see an eye doctor or go to the emergency room.

What should I do if I have indigestion?

Stop drinking coffee, tea, and alcohol

Stop smoking

Take drugstore brand antacids

Elevate the head of your bed six inches

Ask your doctor about prescription drugs (over-the-counter Pepcid and Tagamet are just as expensive and not as effective as prescription drugs)

487

 If you have bright red blood in your stool and you do not have hemorrhoids, see your doctor right away.

488

 If you have trouble gaining weight and frequently feel nervous, warm, and sweaty, you may have an overactive thyroid; see your doctor.

489

 Aspirin is not a good drug for pain relief. (See tip 117.)

490

 Aspirin *is* a good drug to keep your blood from clotting and may protect you against heart attacks. Ask your doctor about it.

491

 The signs of infection are increasing warmth, redness, swelling, pain, and pus.

492

Cuts and infections on your legs and feet are hard to heal. Elevate your feet if you want them to heal faster.

493

Using cocaine can give you a fatal heart attack. If you drink at the same time, your risk is greater. Don't do it.

494

If you knock a tooth out, pick it up by the top part and don't touch the root or bottom part. If it's dirty, rinse it carefully in milk. If you don't have milk, use tap water. Don't scrub or scrape the tooth.

495

If you have a tooth knocked out, save the tooth, and if possible set it back in the socket and bite down gently. (See tip 494.) Time is critical! Go to a dentist or an oral surgeon *immediately*.

496

If you knock out a tooth and can't set it gently back in the socket, it will die in about thirty minutes if it's left out in the air. Holding it carefully, put the tooth in a clean container with fresh, refrigerated milk. It may keep several hours in there. If you can't do this, wrap it tightly in plastic. Don't let it dry out! If you want to save the tooth, find a dentist immediately!

497

Never pet or play with a wild animal such as a raccoon. No matter how cute it looks, it is still wild. If you get bitten, you'll need an unpleasant and expensive series of shots.

498

The reason red wine gives some people headaches is that it contains lots of sulfites, and many people are allergic to them. If sulfites are a problem for you, drink white wine instead.

499

If you often feel unusually happy, energetic, and totally on top of the world and don't feel a need for sleep, see a psychiatrist. If these times are mixed with periods of feeling hopeless, you *must* see a psychiatrist—she can help!

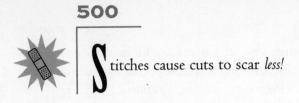

500

Stitches cause cuts to scar *less!*

501

The worst things to burn your eye with are lye products such as drain cleaners, lime for lawns or cement, or ammonia. Acid burns are dangerous, but not as bad.

502

Scabies are a type of tiny insect that live under the skin. They are extremely itchy, especially at night. They often start on the hands and look like little reddish lines. You can catch them from another person or from infected sheets. To get rid of them, see your doctor; you need a prescription.

503

Always try to eat a high fiber diet—it prevents hemorrhoids and constipation, and you may live longer.

504

Don't go to the emergency room and ask for narcotic pain medicine! This includes any medicine with a narcotic ingredient such as Percocet, Vicodan, Tylenol 3, or Tylox. These drugs are federally controlled and emergency room doctors are very reluctant to provide them. If you need pain medicine this potent, ask your regular doctor and make sure you have enough to get through weekends.

505

The extremely contagious herpes virus is the most common cause of genital sores in the United States. If you have sores on your genitals, don't have sex. See your doctor.

506

Neck pain can be extremely painful. Many people have it, and we really don't know what to do about it. Try chiropractic, massage therapy and acupuncture.

507

Skin infection in the hands and face is especially dangerous. If you think you might have it and can't get an appointment with your doctor that day, go to the emergency room.

508

Two drugs for stomach irritation—Pepsid and Tagamet—have recently been released for nonprescription use. They are just as expensive as the prescription drugs and may not be as effective. See your doctor and ask for a more effective prescription.

509

Your best protection against viruses is your own immune system. Take care of it by eating right, getting enough sleep, and keeping your stress level under control.

510

If you are sure you haven't passed any urine for twenty-four hours, see your doctor or go to the emergency room.

511

Smoking can ruin the condition of your skin and make you look almost twice your age.

512

 If you are constipated, try a stool softener called do-cusate sodium before trying a laxative. Take one or two tablets at bedtime and make sure to drink plenty of fluids. Buy the generic brand.

513

 If you are still constipated after taking stool soften-ers, use a laxative such as bisacodyl. The drugstore brand is fine. Drink plenty of fluids.

514

 If a few doses of laxatives haven't helped your con-stipation, try a Fleets enema. Buy them at the drug-store; they are very easy to use. Don't be embarrassed! But if you need to use an enema more than twice, see your doctor.

515

 Gonorrhea and chlamydia are the most common bacterial sexually transmitted diseases. They can be cured with antibiotics. AIDS and herpes are viral and can't be cured.

516

Watch all cuts and burns carefully for signs of infection—increasing redness, warmth, and tenderness, and signs of pus. If your cut becomes infected, see your doctor right away. You need antibiotics.

517

If you hurt your back on the job, tell your boss and let her know that you need light duty for one or two weeks. If she refuses, ask to be sent to a doctor and get a note from him about avoiding heavy work.

518

If you think you have lice or "crabs," look carefully through your pubic hair for the little bugs. Put them into a clear glass and cover it with plastic wrap. Show this to your doctor, and your visit will be faster and less embarrassing than if your doctor has to find the bugs himself.

519

If you injure your elbow and it really hurts to move it, get an x-ray. Broken elbows are very, very painful and usually require a hard cast.

If you have not kept any fluids down for twenty-four hours

If you feel dizzy and weak and vomit up everything you drink

If you have blood or mucus in your diarrhea

If you have a fever higher than 101 degrees

If you also have a continuing pain in your belly that steadily gets worse

If you also have chest pain

520

Carbon monoxide is the leading cause of death due to toxins, and you can't see or smell it. Have your home heating system checked, don't run your car in a closed garage, and if you have headaches, nausea, or dizziness when you drive, have your car exhaust system checked.

521

If you are thinking about getting pregnant, make sure you get lots of folic acid. It's difficult to get enough from your diet. Make sure you get at least 1 milligram a day.

522

If gas bothers you, try a drugstore brand of simethicone. Chew four tablets with plenty of water.

523

If you have chest pain and also feel as if you can't catch your breath, or have nausea, sweating, or fluttering of your heart, go to the emergency room immediately. Take one regular aspirin on the way.

524

If you've been out in the woods and get an expanding, ring-shaped rash, fever, and flulike symptoms a few days later, see your doctor—you may have Lyme disease.

525

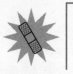

Always keep sterile gauze pads, tape, povidone–iodine, and antibiotic ointment on hand to treat cuts.

526

There is a great prescription antibiotic ointment called Bactroban. Ask your doctor about it.

527

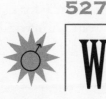

When your penis is partially erect, you are more vulnerable to injury.

528

If you have high blood pressure, don't eat salt. Most of the salt you eat is in packaged or fast foods; cut out these foods first.

What should I do if I stub my toe and it gets black and blue?

———

Ice and elevate the toe

Put cotton between your toes and tape one good toe to the hurt toe

Get an X-ray if it's your big toe and it won't stop hurting

529

 It is easier to sleep in a place that is dark and quiet. If this is impossible, get a sleep mask and ear plugs.

530

 The diet pills sold in the drugstore are just the decongestant phenylpropanolamine, which makes you jittery. If you find this really helps suppress your appetite, it's probably cheaper to buy the same drug in the cold pill section.

531

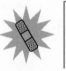 If you step on a nail, make sure you get a tetanus shot, unless you've had one within the past five years. Clean the cut, elevate your foot, and watch carefully for signs of infection. Most puncture wounds won't get infected, but it might. If it does, see your doctor right away!

532

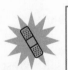 Sometimes when you step on a nail a piece of sock or dirt gets into your foot. You can get a very nasty bone infection from this. If you feel that there is something still in your foot, or you feel any signs of infection, such as redness, pain, or swelling, see your doctor immediately.

533

 If your sinuses are always blocked, you've taken many courses of antibiotics, and it always seems to return, see an ear, nose, and throat specialist. Chronic sinusitis is no fun.

534

 If your arm or leg is in a cast, do not put anything inside it to scratch your skin with. You could develop a terrible infection.

535

 Caffeine is an upper. If you feel jumpy or have trouble sleeping, don't drink caffeine!

536

 People who die from an overdose of alcohol usually choke on their own vomit. This is an awful way to die. Don't abuse alcohol.

537

If you are stung on or around the eye by an insect, the area will probably swell a lot—you'll notice this especially after sleeping. Take a tea bag and steep it in warm water. After it has cooled a bit, lay it on your eye and relax for half an hour. This should take down the swelling. Do this as often as necessary.

538

If you have trouble getting lubricated enough to enjoy sex, buy some oil made especially for that purpose. Don't be embarrassed—this is a very common problem.

539

When you get your eyes checked, make sure your doctor checks for glaucoma. This is an especially common eye disease in older people.

540

If you feel terribly stressed and don't feel you have time to relax, each time you go to the bathroom or get in your car, spend a few minutes just noticing your breathing.

541

If your newly pierced ears get infected, and it spreads to the rest of your ear, your ear could become deformed. See your doctor immediately.

542

If the rims of your eyelids and your eyelashes get red and have greasy, scaly stuff on them, wash them gently but thoroughly with baby shampoo until it goes away.

543

If the rims of your eyelids are very red and your eyelashes have lots of *honey-colored* crusts on them, see an eye doctor.

544

If you have red eyes with a crusty discharge, you probably have conjunctivitis. If your eyelids and a larger area around your eye are also red, swollen, and painful, and you have a fever, see an eye doctor or go to the emergency room right away.

545

If you come in from the cold and your fingers and toes feel numb and painful, do *not* put them under hot water or in front of a fire. Tuck your fingers into your armpits. Put on warm, dry clothes and wait. If you still have pain in several hours or get blisters or broken skin, see your doctor.

546

If you have had sex without using a condom and are worried about getting gonorrhea or chlamydia, see your doctor. You can often take two doses of antibiotics and not need to worry.

547

When you are in the hospital, try to keep a log of all the medicines they give you, the tests performed, and all your doctor visits. Then when you check your bill you'll have something solid to refer to.

548

Acupuncture can help you quit smoking.

549

Cold sores on your lips are caused by a virus related to the one that causes genital herpes. If you have a cold sore, wash your hands after touching your lips and before touching your genitals.

550

If you go to a psychotherapist and plan to bill it to your insurance company, ask the therapist not to use the diagnosis of "depression." This may lessen your chances of getting health and disability insurance in the future.

551

If you get ingrown toenails, try cutting them straight across and then cutting a V shape right in the center. Sometimes this will make the nail grow toward the center instead of growing into the sides.

552

If you miss a period, you can try a home pregnancy test after it's a week late. If the test is positive, see your doctor or go to a clinic. If the test is negative, wait another week and try again. If it's still negative and you haven't gotten your period, see your doctor.

553

If you jam a finger playing sports, make sure you can straighten the finger out completely and can also make a tight fist. Then ice it, elevate it, and try to keep it stable using a slightly curved splint from the drugstore. See your doctor if you can't extend it out fully or if you think it might be broken.

554

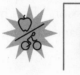

Green tea and many herbal teas contain caffeine.

555

The mouth of a cat is very dirty. If you are bitten, wash the bite carefully with povidone–iodine, apply some antibiotic ointment, and cover it. Make sure the cat has had a rabies shot. Then see your doctor or go to the emergency room—*cat bites typically get infected.*

556

Find out how the medical coverage for your auto insurance works. That's the last thing you'll want to deal with when you need to visit the emergency room after a car accident.

557

If you have significant bleeding from your vagina after having sex, go to the emergency room.

558

If you are traveling in a poorly developed country, don't eat anything that you can't peel or that hasn't been thoroughly cooked. Make sure to avoid anything that might have been washed, such as lettuce or grapes. Don't forget to avoid sauces such as salsa that haven't been cooked. Do not believe people when they tell you the food or water is safe. Spending your vacation bent over a toilet is not fun.

559

Your lips need sun protection—*use it.*

When should I go to the emergency room with a head injury?

If you lost consciousness for any length of time

If you are vomiting uncontrollably

If your balance is off or you feel lethargic or unable to stay awake

If you have any numbness in your hands and feet

If you have any neck pain

If you have abnormal vision or hearing

560

If you get a dark blue bruise under a fingernail, there's probably blood under it. Sterilize a large needle in a flame, clean the fingernail and needle with some povidone–iodine, then slowly rotate the needle into the nail over the area that looks the bluest. This will not hurt! The blood will come out through the needle hole. Push gently on the nail to get all the blood out. Then put some antibiotic ointment on the nail and cover and elevate it. Watch for signs of infection. If the pain increases, see your doctor.

561

After you eat asparagus, your urine will probably smell funny. Don't worry, *it's normal.*

562

If you have distinct periods of extreme nervousness that accompany sensations such as a pounding heart, tingling of your fingers, or shortness of breath, you may be having panic attacks. See a psychiatrist! This can be treated.

563

A steam burn can be much worse than a burn from dry heat.

564

If you hit your head but didn't lose consciousness, you may still feel strange for several days. Minor dizziness, headache, feeling "spacey," and nausea are common problems after a head injury. If you have these problems for more than a few days, or they are severe, see your doctor.

565

Genital warts are very common and easy to transmit to sexual partners. They are also difficult to treat. See your doctor if you see wartlike sores on your genital area.

566

Caffeine makes you urinate more. If you have diarrhea or need fluids, don't drink caffeine.

What is the best medicine for pain if I have a bruise or muscle sprain?

If you don't have stomach problems, use ibuprofen

If you have stomach problems or ulcers, use acetaminophen

Use ice

567

If you cut your lip on the inside and it stops bleeding with some direct pressure, it probably doesn't need stitches. Try not to irritate the cut and check it the next morning.

568

Sometimes a diaphragm can cause pain and a burning feeling when you urinate. If you feel these symptoms after using your diaphragm, see your gynecologist. You may need a smaller size.

569

If you do get sick while on vacation, drink as much bottled water as you can. If you are vomiting, wait twenty minutes, then keep trying to take small sips. Don't take medicine for diarrhea unless you must.

570

If you have a strained neck, don't use one of those big white collars unless it really makes you feel better. These collars *generally* make your neck more stiff and painful.

571

If you're a woman, you are five times more likely than a man to break your hip. This is because women often don't get enough calcium, and their bones get weak. Take your calcium pills!

572

The human mouth is packed with germs. A human bite can be dangerous. If you get bitten by another person, wash the bite out with povidone–iodine and go to the emergency room right away.

573

The worst thing about a human bite is the possibility of getting hepatitis or AIDS. If you get bitten, try to find out if the person has ever had hepatitis or has AIDS (HIV) virus, which *can* be spread by saliva. (This is not likely, but it *is* possible.)

574

If you get bitten by someone, go to the emergency room. You will need a booster shot to help protect you against hepatitis and information about how and when to get tested for AIDS (HIV) virus. Human bites often get infected, so you must get antibiotics and a tetanus shot.

575

If you are not planning on having a child in the next five years, ask your doctor about the birth control method called Norplant. Tiny capsules, which you can barely feel, are placed in your arm. If you change your mind and want to have a child, you can ask your doctor to take them out. Make sure you consult a gynecologist.

576

The creams that claim to help sprains don't work. All they do is heat up the skin. If you feel better after using them it's only because you massaged them in. Instead, massage with an ordinary skin cream, then use ice.

577

If your nose and sinuses are always blocked, you can use a steroid nasal spray. This really works and can make you much more comfortable. Ask your doctor about it.

578

Sunscreens wear off. Put them on every three hours. If you've been swimming, put more on when you get out of the water.

579

Strong tea and coffee have about the same amount of caffeine per cup.

580

If you are in the sun, wear a sunscreen with both UVA and UVB protection. It should list those on the bottle or say "broad spectrum."

581

Breathing problems are true emergencies. If you have trouble breathing, go to the emergency room.

582

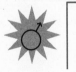

If you have an erection that is not from being aroused sexually, and it will not go away, go to the emergency room. This is called priapism.

583

If your contact lenses scratch your eye, don't tape your eye closed. See your eye doctor and don't wear your contacts for at least a week.

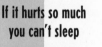

When should I go to the emer-gency room with an earache?

If it hurts so much you can't sleep

If you are a dia-betic and it hurts when you tug on your ear

It you also experi-ence a loss of hearing

If you have discharge

584

If you are a man, have had unprotected sex, and three to five days afterwards you have real pain when you urinate and lots of yellowish discharge from your penis, see your doctor. You probably have gonorrhea.

585

If you are a man, have had unprotected sex, and about a week or so later notice a slight pain when you urinate and a clear or milky discharge from your penis mainly in the mornings, you may have a sexually transmitted disease called chlamydia. See your doctor.

586

Caffeine is an addictive drug. If you stop drinking it suddenly, you may get a withdrawal headache. If you plan to stop, do it slowly.

587

If you are going to bed soon after getting a burn, crush some fresh onion and lay it over the burn. Cover it well with a Band-Aid and go to bed. The burn should feel better in the morning. (See tip 80.)

588

If you cut off a piece of your finger or toe, apply pressure firmly to stop the bleeding and elevate it. Then wrap the piece that was cut off in a clean plastic bag and put it on top of an ice pack that is wrapped in a towel. Go to the emergency room immediately. If you have a choice, pick a hospital that is a teaching center or has a medical school attached to it—you have a better chance of finding a highly-trained surgeon there.

589

If your toenails look very yellowed and thicker than normal, you may have fungus under them. If this goes untreated for very long, it's almost impossible to cure. See a podiatrist!

590

If you get a cut on your scalp, it's probably going to bleed like crazy. Don't worry—apply direct, constant pressure to stop the bleeding. Wash it with povidone–iodine, dry, and leave it alone for three to four days. That means don't wash your hair! If it stops bleeding, is less than an inch long, and is not gaping open, it probably doesn't need stitches. The scalp heals very fast.

What should I do if I can't sleep at night?

Cut out all caffeine after 2:00 P.M.

Stop drinking alcohol

Use a sleep mask and earplugs

Take one generic (drugstore brand) Benedryl at bedtime

Start a sleep routine

591

If you get bitten by an animal or a person and haven't had a tetanus shot in the past five years, you need to get one as soon as possible.

592

Find a moisturizer with sunscreen and use it every day.

593

Smoking causes heart disease, cancer, and many other illnesses. Secondhand smoke is almost as bad. If you must smoke, don't do it around your kids!

594

Before you leave on vacation, ask your doctor for some antibiotics to take in case you get sick.

595

To remove a tick, pour mineral oil or alcohol over it to kill it. Then slowly and carefully remove it with tweezers, making sure you get the head out.

596

If you have lots of moles, see a skin doctor who will monitor them for you.

597

Hydrocortisone 1 percent cream is the only drug-store anti-itch cream that works. Buy the generic. Benadryl cream and the other antihistamine creams are not effective—don't bother with them.

598

If you are taking any type of prescription medicine and you notice a rash, stop taking the medicine and call your doctor. The rash may take a week or more to go away. Take diphenhydramine for itching.

599

If you know you have an allergy to bee stings (if you have problems breathing after being stung), you should always carry an "Epi-pen." This device allows you to immediately inject yourself with the right medicine. If you need one, ask your doctor for a prescription, then see an allergist for a long-term cure.

What should I be prepared to tell the doctor when I go to the emergency room?

How long you've had the problem

If it is connected with any other complaints

If you've had it before

(continued)

600

Quitting smoking is one of the hardest things you may ever have to do. To make it easier, first cut down to just the number of cigarettes you can't live without—for most people this is about six or seven a day. After about a week, take the cigarettes you have left, run them under water, then throw them out. The first three days will be *hell*, but you will survive!

601

If you're trying to quit smoking, chew on plastic coffee stirrers, gum, or hard candy. Calculate the amount of money you'll save and buy yourself a present. It's helpful to be in touch with a support group of some kind.

602

If you've quit smoking, it's crucial to never smoke another cigarette.

603

If you can't quit smoking on your own, talk to your doctor about other options such as acupuncture, hypnosis, or the nicotine patch.

604

Don't be afraid to ask your doctor about *any* medical issue you don't understand.

605

Americans think illness means weakness and they are reluctant to admit to being sick. Everyone gets sick. If you feel ill, stay home and take good care of yourself—your long-term health will be better.

What makes it better, and what makes it worse

If you've tried any treatments and whether or not they worked

The name of your doctor and her phone number

The names of all your medicines (keep a list)

Glossary

Acetaminophen The ingredient in Tylenol and most aspirin-free pain medicine. It's a pain reliever that is safe for people with stomach problems but not for people with liver problems or those who drink more than three ounces of alcohol a day.

Advil A brand-name medicine that contains ibuprofen.

Aluminum Hydroxide A common ingredient in antacids. It can produce constipation.

Anesthetic A class of drugs that numbs, usually applied to the skin or mouth when used in nonprescription medications.

Antibiotic A drug that kills bacteria. In over-the-counter medicines it's usually found in ointments for use on the skin. Use a generic "triple" ointment—this has three kinds of antibiotics and is more likely to work.

Anticholinergic A class of drugs often used for motion sickness or stomach cramps. It works on your nervous system making you sleepy, your mouth dry, and your vision blurry. Don't use it if you have prostate problems or glaucoma.

Antihistamine A class of drugs that controls allergic reactions, such as hives and hay fever. Over-the-counter antihistamines can make you sleepy.

Anusol A brand-name medication that comes as a cream or suppository. It's useful for hemorrhoids and contains pramoxine.

Aspirin   A familiar drug for pain, but not very effective for pain control and hard on the stomach. It may be useful for heart attacks.

Attapulgite   This is the active ingredient in drugs like Kaopectate. It slows down your gut when you have diarrhea. Buy the generic brand.

Bacitracin   An antibiotic ointment used on the skin for cuts and burns.

Benadryl   The brand name for diphenhydramine, the most common antihistamine.

Benzocaine   A local anesthetic, often used directly on the skin.

Benzoyl Peroxide   A drying agent, often used in gels and soaps for pimples and acne. It works well and can be used twice a day. If your skin gets very red and irritated, use it less often.

Beta Carotene   An "antioxidant" compound, found in foods and vitamins, which may protect against some types of cancer.

Bisacodyl   A stimulant laxative that works directly on the gut. It's stronger than fiber or vegetable laxatives.

Bismuth (Subsalicylate)   A drug that soaks up fluid in the gut, so it helps diarrhea. It's the ingredient in Pepto Bismol. Don't take it if you have a severe aspirin allergy. Remember, it will make your stool dark black.

Brompheniramine Maleate A common antihistamine. It makes you sleepy.

Burrows Solution   Used as a fluid to soak rashes with blisters, such as poison ivy, poison oak, and chicken pox.

Caffeine   A stimulant found in coffee, tea, and soda. It can make you jumpy, cause heart skips, and give you insomnia.

Calamine   A lotion used to dry out the blisters in itchy rashes. Burrows solution works better, but calamine is portable. Calamine does not lessen the itch.

Calcium   A mineral that comes combined with either carbonate or chloride in drugstore supplements. All women should take 1,200 milligrams of elemental calcium a day.

Carbamide Peroxide   A chemical that helps to dissolve ear wax. Use it with a bulb ear syringe. Buy the generic.

Cascara   A stimulant laxative that works directly on the gut.

Charcoal   Charcoal comes in a liquid and in capsules. Keep some in the house and give a dose if someone swallows something poisonous. Don't use if lye is swallowed. Call poison control immediately!

Cholorpheniramine Maleate
A common antihistamine—it makes you sleepy.

Clotrimazole   A good cream to use on the skin for fungal infections.

Coal Tar   An ingredient in dandruff shampoos that is stronger than selenium, the chemical in Selsun Blue.

Codeine Phosphate   A narcotic medicine used for pain and in prescription cough medicines. It can cause nausea and constipation.

Colace   The brand name for docusate sodium, a stool softener. It's can also be used in liquid form for dissolving ear wax.

Colloidal Oatmeal   The ingredient in Aveeno, it soothes itchy skin when used in a bath.

Cyclizine Hydrochloride   An antihistamine ingredient used to control motion sickness. The drug meclizine is much better. If you are pregnant, don't use either drug.

Decongestant   A class of drugs that decrease swelling and open your nose and sinuses. It may make you feel jumpy.

Dexbrompheniramine Maleate
A common antihistamine.

Dextromethorphan Hydrobromide
The most common nonprescription cough suppressant.

Dibucaine   A local anesthetic used in hemorrhoid cream. It's not as effective as pramoxine.

Dimenhydrinate   An antihistamine used in Dramamine for motion sickness. It makes you sleepy.

Diphenhydramine Citrate/ Diphenhydramine Hydrochloride   A common, very safe, and effective antihistamine used in most of the sleep and allergy medicines. The brand name is Benadryl.

Domeboro's Solution   A brand name for Burrows solution. It dries blisters from poison ivy, chicken pox, and shingles.

Docusate Calcium/Docusate Potassium/Ducisate Sodium   Common stool softeners. They're not actually laxatives, but soften the consistency of stool.

Emertrol   A brand-name medicine for nausea that is basically a sugar syrup. Don't use this if you are diabetic, but it won't hurt you otherwise.

Epsom Salts   A solution for soaking infected areas.

Equalactin   A brand name product that claims to be good for Irritable Bowl Syndrome. This stuff is just fiber; try generic fiber supplements instead. If you really have irritable bowel syndrome they may make you worse, but you can try them.

Erythromycin   A common antibiotic which should not be taken at the same time as Seldane or Hismanal, two prescription antihistamines. Don't take it with theophylline or Nizoral either.

Expectorant   A class of drugs that helps liquefy thick mucus from your nose, sinuses, and chest.

Ferrous Fumarate/Ferrous Gluconate/Ferrous Sulfate   These are all iron supplements.

Folic Acid   A very important vitamin during pregnancy. It is included in most multivitamin pills.

Griseofulvin   A drug taken orally for fungal infections. It should never be taken at the same time as Seldane or Hismanal.

Guaifenesin   A common expectorant in cough and cold medicines. Make sure to take it with plenty of liquids.

Hismanal   An excellent prescription antihistamine that doesn't make you sleepy. Don't take it with erythromycin or griseofulvin or antidepressants such as Prozac.

HCL or Hydrochloride   A chemical ending that you should generally ignore, as long as the drug name before it is the drug in which you are interested.

Hydrocortisone Cream   An anti-inflammatory cream used on the skin for itching. It's the best drug available over the counter. The strongest is 1 percent; the weakest is 0.5 percent (usually labeled hydrocortisone 10 and 5). Don't use it if you think the area is infected.

Hydrogen Peroxide   Good for dissolving blood and cleaning cuts on the skin.

Ibuprofen   The main ingredient in Advil, Motrin, Nuprin, etc. It's an anti-inflammatory and is excellent for sprains and menstrual cramps. It's the most popular drug of this type sold over the counter. If you have ulcers or a sensitive stomach be careful with this drug. Don't take it if you are allergic to aspirin. A good dose is 600 milligrams (usually three pills), every eight hours. Take it with food.

Ipecac   A medicine that makes you vomit quickly and repeatedly. Don't use it if someone swallows lye or something such as gasoline, which will do more harm if it comes back up. Charcoal is a safer bet if you are not sure, but call poison control right away!

Iron   A dietary supplement. Don't use too much of this until further research clarifies if it is harmful.

Isopropyl Alcohol   Often used for cleaning the skin, it does not kill bacteria very well. It does clean off dirt and grime.

Kaopectate   An excellent drug for diarrhea caused by food poisoning.

Lactase   The natural substance that digests lactose, the sugar found in milk products. If you have trouble digesting foods such as milk, ice cream, and cheese, use the drugstore brand pills that supply this substance.

Lidocaine Hydrochloride
A common local anesthetic often used in first aid sprays. It's better to use hydrocortisone if you have sunburn, and antibiotic ointment if you have a cut.

Loperamide Hydrochloride   An excellent drug for diarrhea. But if you have food poisoning, use Kaopectate.

Magnesium Carbonate/
Magnesium Chloride/
Magnesium Gluconate/
Magnesium Hydroxide/
Magnesium Oxide   All of these are forms of magnesium—they act as an antacid in the gut. They can give you diarrhea if you take too much.

Meclizine   An antihistamine that is excellent for motion sickness. It will make you sleepy and dry out your mouth.

Miconazole Nitrate   A good drug used in creams for fungus that grows on the skin and causes athletes foot and jock itch.

Motrin   A brand name medicine that contains ibuprofen.

Naproxen   The ingredient in the brand-name drug Aleve. It is a good drug for sprains, menstrual cramps, and generalized pain, although it can be hard on the stomach. You can take up to six pills a day with food. There is currently no generic form of this drug available for use without a prescription. Don't combine this drug with aspirin.

Narcotic   The general name for pain control drugs that have tranquilizing effects. These drugs can also be habit forming.

Neomycin Sulfate   An antibiotic; one of the usual ingredients in antibiotic ointments.

Nonoxynol-9   A drug that kills sperm. It is used in contraceptive creams and condoms and may cause irritation to the vagina.

Nuprin   A brand-name medicine that contains ibuprofen.

Oxymetazoline Hydrochloride
The ingredient in long lasting nasal sprays. It works pretty well if you follow the instructions exactly.

My advice is to skip these sprays. (See tip 109.)

Phenylephrine Hydrochloride A decongestant; it clears up your nose but can make you jumpy.

Phenylpropanolamine Hydrochloride A decongestant generally used in non-prescription diet pills. It makes you very jumpy and occasionally causes you to forget you're hungry.

Polymyxin Sulfate An antibiotic— one of the ingredients in antibiotic ointments.

Potassium or Sodium Bicarbonate An antacid contained in products such as Alka Seltzer. It causes you to belch, which might make you feel better. If you really have acid indigestion or heartburn, don't use this; use plain antacids instead.

Potassium Nitrate The main ingredient in toothpastes for sensitive teeth. It works quite well.

Povidone–Iodine Sold in a 10 percent solution. It's the best thing for cleaning cuts and scratches. It's also sold under the brand name Betadine.

Pramoxine The best cream for hemorrhoids. Look for it as an ingredient in drugstore brand creams.

Pseudoephedrine Hydrochloride The most common decongestant. It tends to make you jittery, but it's very good for opening your stuffy nose. Don't use it if you have high blood pressure.

Psychopharmacology A medical specialty that deals chiefly with psychiatric medicines.

Psyllium The type of fiber contained in most of the name-brand bulking agents such as Metamucil. This product is good for you: It makes your bowels work faster and may help you live longer. Buy the generic.

Pyrantel Pamoate This product is quite expensive, but it's the best drug for pinworms. You don't need a prescription.

Salicylic Acid A type of drying agent usually put in soaps for acne. It's also used in gels and solutions for dissolving warts.

Seldane   A fairly weak prescription antihistamine that should not be taken at the same time as erythromycin or griseofulvin or an antidepressant such as Prozac.

Selenium Sulfide   The ingredient that makes some dandruff shampoos work.

Simethicone   The best thing for gas. Take it with plenty of fluids and chew it well.

Steroids   The common name for a family of very strong anti-inflammatory drugs. Steroids are used in many different prescription medicines.

Theophylline   An outdated drug for asthma, sold as Primatene tablets. Don't use this drug—it's been replaced by much better ones. Ask your doctor about a prescription for inhaled steroids.

Tolnafate   A medicine for a fungus such as athletes foot; it's not as good as miconazole.

Triprolidine Hydrochloride
A strong antihistamine. It makes you very sleepy but it's excellent for itchy, allergic rashes. If you buy it combined with a decongestant, you may be able to stay awake.

Trolamine Salicylate   A drug used in anesthetic creams for the skin. Do not use this—it can be dangerous.

Undecylenic Acid   A drug used in Desenex antifungal cream; it's also known as zinc undecylenate. Do not use either drug.

Zinc Oxide   An ingredient in thick creams used for total sunscreen and diaper irritation. It works very well.

123 Paste   After checking with your doctor, your pharmacist can make this for diaper rash or any skin that needs protection from urine or other irritants. It's 1 part aluminum acetate, 2 parts aquaphor, 3 parts zinc oxide.

Index